Clinical Film Viewing Series

RESPIRATORY SYSTEM

Dedication

I dedicate this book to my wife, Lois

Clinical Film Viewing Series

Series Editor: Paul R. Goddard

RESPIRATORY SYSTEM

Paul R. Goddard, BSC, MB BS, MD, DMRD, FRCR
Consultant Radiologist, Bristol Royal Infirmary
Clinical Lecturer, Bristol University

With a Foreword by
Professor E. R. Davies CBE
Professor of Radiodiagnosis, University of Bristol

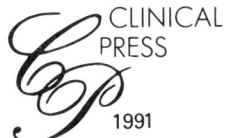

CLINICAL PRESS
1991

© **Copyright Clinical Press Limited.** 1991

All rights reserved. No part of this publication may be reproduced, stored in a retrieval system, transmitted in any form or by any means, electronic, mechanical, photocopying, recording or otherwise, without the prior permission of the Copyright Owner.

Published by:
Clinical Press Limited,
Registered Office, Redland Green Farm, Redland Green,
Redland, BRISTOL, BS6 7HF.

British Library Cataloguing in Publication Data
Goddard Paul R.
 Respiratory system.
 1. Man. Respiratory system. Diagnosis.
 I. Title II. Series
 616.20047572

ISBN 1-85457-014-5

Produced by G.P.E. Ltd
Clevedon, Avon BS21 7TG

Typeset by:
Apek Typesetters
Avon House, Blackfriars Road,
Nailsea, Bristol BS19 2DJ

Printed by:
Albany House Ltd.
Coleshill, Warwickshire

Contents

Foreword	vii
Introduction	viii
Acknowledgements	viii
Eighty Diagnostic Exercises	1
Index	162

Foreword

by **Professor E. R. Davies** CBE

The archetype of medical teaching is the illustrated case. It has been the backbone of all the ward rounds and radiological tutorials that we have ever attended. As the body of radiological knowledge increased, systematic collection of data in comprehensive textbooks became necessary and so did the need for systematic lecture programmes. The received wisdom from these sources deserved to be validated and enlarged by serious research and the robust health of our journals attest the quality of such research.

The student of radiology—whatever his seniority or professional persuasion—thus has comprehensive data resource. And yet the day-to-day commerce of clinical radiology trades in the art of applying this information to specific case problems. This art can only be acquired by supervised practice and experience. The importance of acquiring it is emphasised in the structure of the Final FRCR Examination and its international equivalents which contain a film reporting component carrying considerable weight. Non-radiologists require a working knowledge of the application of radiology to their discipline and this is recognised by the inclusion of radiographic interpretation in the Membership Examination for the Royal College of Physicians.

Dr Goddard has many years of experience as a University Lecturer and as teacher to undergraduates and postgraduates in radiology and other clinical disciplines. His most valuable teaching experiences come from his involvement with computed tomography and magnetic resonance. He tackled both these advanced techniques when they were absolutely new and his personal mastery of them is reflected in his skill for introducing them into his teaching programme.

The teaching programme contained in this new volume of the series reflects a wide range of interests, interpretive skills and an enthusiasm for communication—essential teaching attributes.

E. Rhys Davies
Professor of Radiodiagnosis
University of Bristol

Introduction

Many of the postgraduate examinations now include X-ray interpretation which may be presented as a slide show or as a film-viewing session. In addition radiographs and other imaging modalities are used ubiquitously in the 'viva' section of most major postgraduate examinations including those of the American Boards and of professional societies and universities world wide.

In a typical examination, candidates are presented with a film and are presented with a minimum of relevant clinical information. They are then asked to give a written or oral report together with a sensible list for the differential diagnosis.

It is the intention of this series of books on *Clinical Film Viewing* to assist the candidates in preparing themselves for this process. Each book examines a particular system or technique and promotes the readers own self-questioning about the films presented.

The *Clinical Film Viewing Series* provides a unique opportunity for self-assessment and learning in all the modern modalities of diagnostic imaging.

Paul R. Goddard

Acknowledgements

I would like to acknowledge the assistance of my radiological and clinical colleagues without which this book would not have been possible.

The cases were investigated at the Bristol Royal Infirmary, the Bristol Radiotherapy Centre, the Bristol General Hospital, the Bristol MRI Centre and the Bupa-Glen Hospital.

Case 1

Sophie, 58, was seized by a sudden severe chest pain extending into the back. Unequal pulses were detected. Her chest X-ray is shown (*Fig.* 1).

Report on the chest X-ray.

Suggest further investigations.

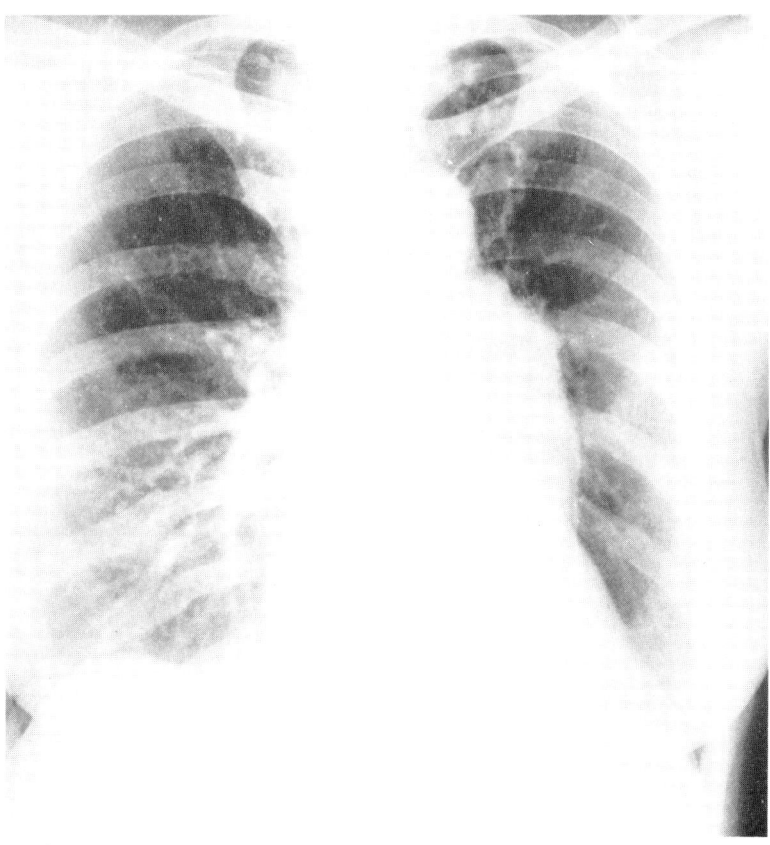

Fig. 1

Answer: Case 1

The heart size and shape are normal. There is, however, marked widening of the mediastinum immediately above the heart with an opacity superimposed on the left hilum. The lung fields appear clear.

In view of the clinical history and chest X-ray appearances, the possibility of a dissecting aneurysm of the aorta must be considered. It is the practice in Bristol to investigate such patients initially with rapid sequential CT scans using a bolus of intravenous contrast medium. The CT scan is shown (*Fig. 2*).

The main pulmonary trunk, ascending aorta, right atrium and left atrium are clearly shown opacified by contrast media. There is widening of the descending aorta and an intimal flap and false lumen are demonstrated.

In the absence of abnormality of the ascending aorta, the descending thoracic aortic dissection is treated conservatively. If the ascending aorta is involved it may be important, with regard to surgical management, to assess whether or not there is aortic regurgitation and involvement of coronary arteries.

Regurgitation can be demonstrated by Doppler echocardiography but good visualization of the coronary arteries does require angiography. MRI is another technique that is being used to demonstrate aortic dissection, regurgitation and involvement of coronary arteries.

(See also in the same series, Hartnell, *Film Viewing in the Cardiovascular System*, Clinical Press).

A flow chart for the diagnosis of a mediastinal mass is shown (*Fig. 3*). (This case is presented by courtesy of Professor E. R. Davies.)

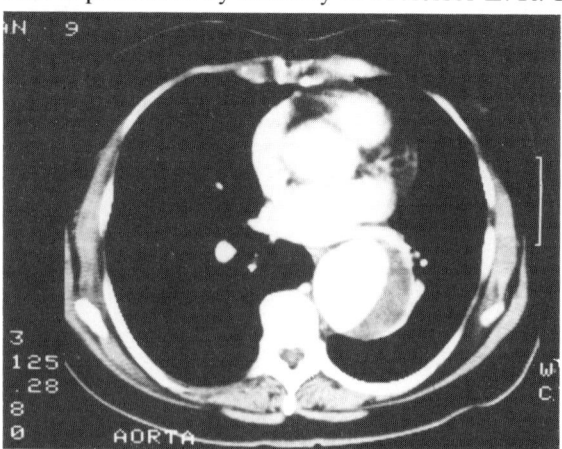

Fig. 2

Case 3

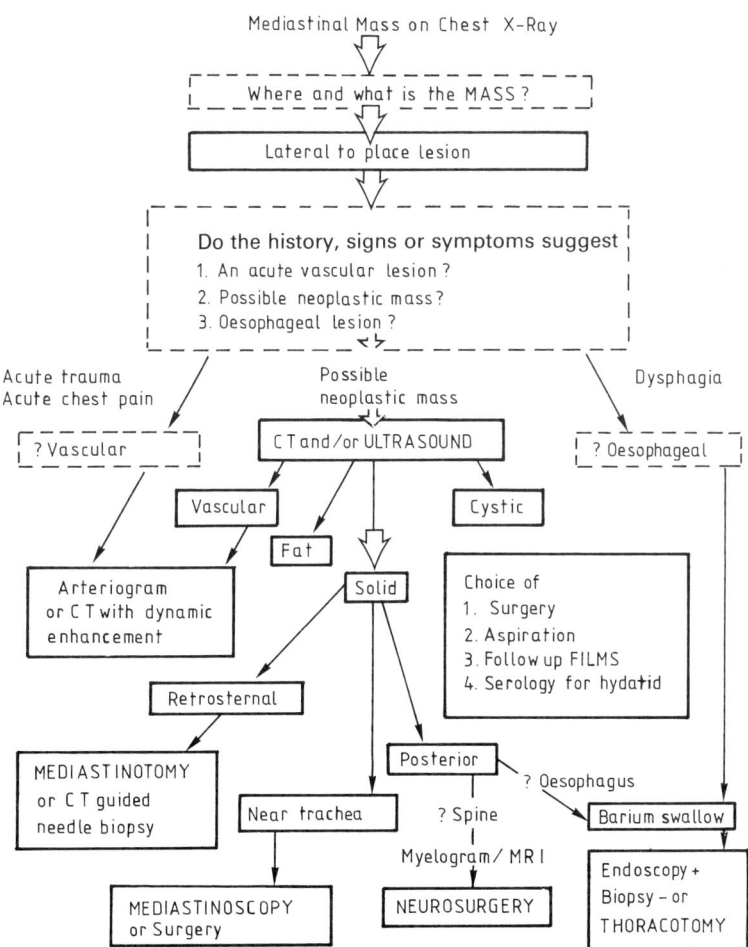

Fig. 3

Case 2

A woman, aged 25, presented with generalized malaise and had the following chest X-ray (*Fig.* 4).

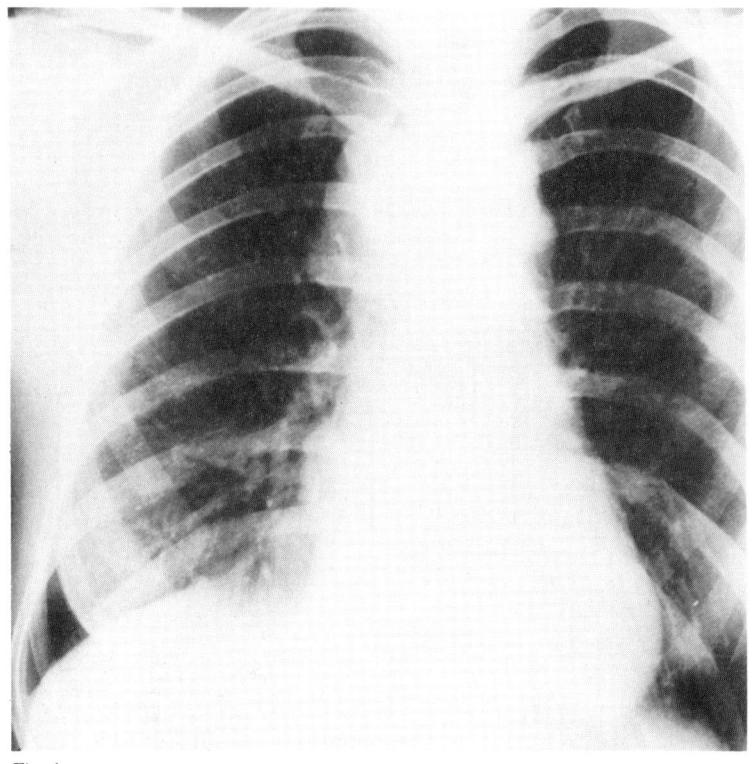

Fig. 4

Answer: Case 2

The heart size and shape are normal. There is marked widening of the mediastinum. In the absence of history of acute onset the most likely cause is lymphoma. Careful examination for peripheral nodes is essential and CT may be indicated as the next radiological investigation.

Examination of the neck revealed cervical nodes and biopsy showed nodular sclerosing Hodgkin's disease. In view of the diagnosis, CT of chest, abdomen and pelvis were obtained for staging purposes. A repeat chest X-ray after chemotherapy showed considerable improvement (*Fig.* 5).

The investigation of mediastinal widening depends to a large extent on the presentation. A table of causes of mediastinal widening is included below.

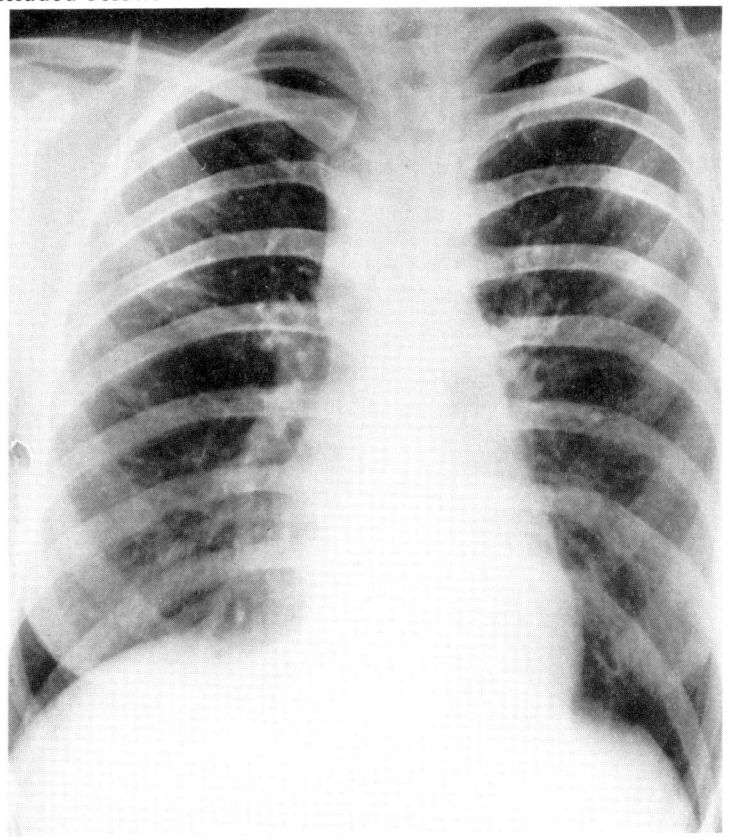

Fig. 5

Table 2.1. Causes of a mediastinal mass

Masses arising anywhere in the mediastinum
1. Lymphadenopathy (secondary carcinoma, lymphoma, sarcoidosis, tuberculosis)
2. Lipoma
3. Fibroma
4. Vascular origin: aneurysm, anomalous vessels, haematoma
5. Abscess

Superior mediastinum
1. Thyroid goitre
2. Pharyngeal pouch
3. Masses that arise anywhere in the mediastinum

Anterior mediastinum
1. Retrosternal thyroid
2. Thymoma and thymic cyst
3. Tetratodermoid
4. Pericardial and pleuropericardial cyst
5. Morgagni hernia
6. Masses that arise anywhere in the mediastinum

Middle mediastinum
1. Cardiac abnormalities
2. Bronchogenic cyst
3. Masses arising anywhere in the mediastinum

Posterior mediastinum
1. Oesophageal abnormality—achalasia, carcinoma, hiatus hernia
2. Aortic aneurysm and other masses that arise anywhere in the mediastinum
3. Neurogenic tumours—including neurofibroma and meningocoele
4. Spinal and paraspinal lesions
5. Bochdalek hernia

Lesions 'simulating' a mediastinal mass
Pulmonary, pleural or chest wall masses abutting the mediastinum

Reference
Goddard P. R. (1987) *Diagnostic Imaging of the Chest.* London, Churchill-Livingstone, pp. 132–133.

Case 3

A man, aged 70, presented with occasional chest pair (*Fig.* 6).

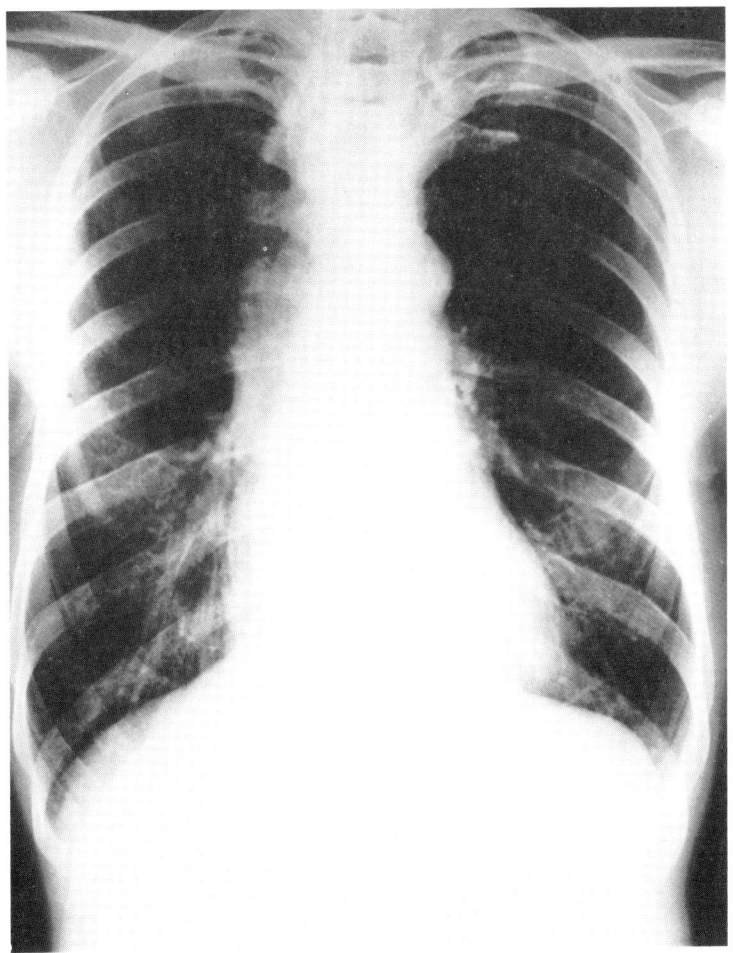

Fig. 6

Answer: Case 3

The chest X-ray shows mediastinal widening with an unusual 'double' shadow affecting the right heart border and mediastinum. There is no stomach bubble visible under the left hemidiaphragm.

The appearances suggest an abnormality affecting the oesophagus—either achalasia, scleroderma or post-surgery. In the absence of any previous history a barium swallow was performed. This showed smooth tapering of the lower end of the oesophagus due to achalasia.

Case 4

A man, aged 29, was brought into the Accident and Emergency Department following a road traffic accident. He complained of chest pain. Two supine AP films three hours apart are shown (*Figs.* 7, 8).

Report on the films and recommend further investigations.

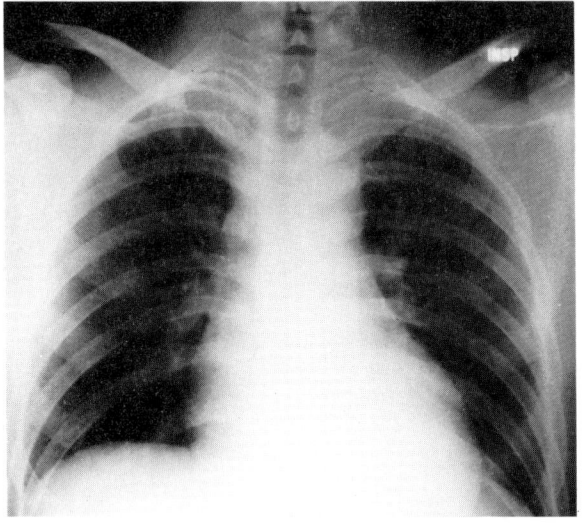

Fig. 7

Case 4

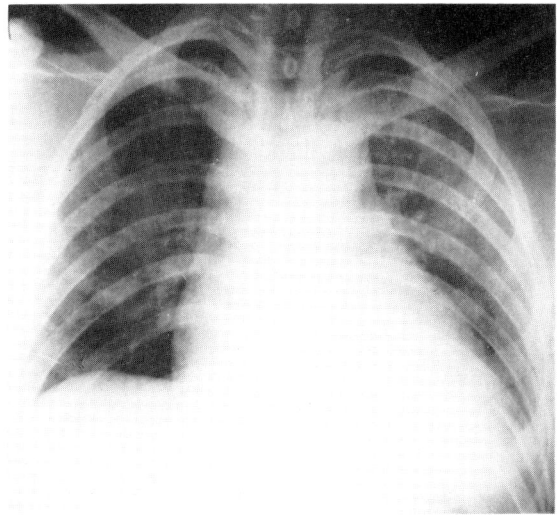

Fig. 8

Answer: Case 4

Allowing for projection the initial AP film shows a normal-sized heart and no lung lesion.

The later film shows a relatively poor inspiration, the mediastinum appears widened, there is increased density of the left hemithorax and slight deviation of the trachea to the right.

The later appearances could be the result of poor inspiratory effort but a repeat film showed no improvement. In view of the history, trauma to the aorta or great vessels must be suspected.

An aortogram was performed (*Fig.* 9) and this shows dilatation of the proximal part of the descending thoracic aorta extending down to an oblique linear radiolucency within the lumen of the aorta at the level of the isthmus. Below this level the density of the contrast medium is decreased. The left internal mammary artery is seen medial to the descending thoracic aorta as a parallel vertical opacity.

The appearances are those of a partial traumatic rupture of the aorta.

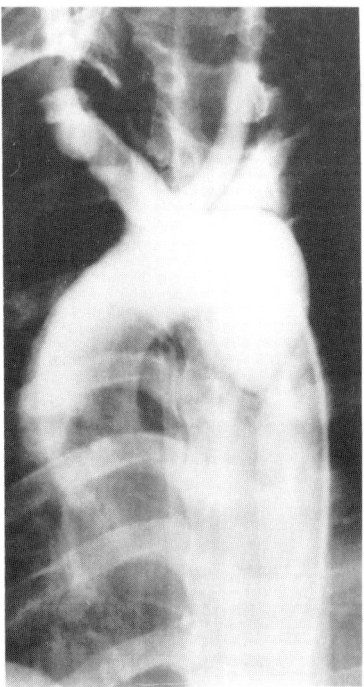

Fig. 9

Comment

Eighty-five per cent of patients with traumatic aortic rupture die before reaching hospital. In the remaining 15% the rupture is partial and is contained by the adventitia and surrounding connective tissue. The widening of the mediastinum in these patients is usually due to a haematoma from venous bleeding rather that arterial.

(This case is presented by courtesy of Professor E. R. Davies.)

Case 5

Annette, aged 39, was involved in a severe road traffic accident. Her chest X-ray is shown (*Fig.* 10).

Report on the chest X-ray, suggest possible diagnoses and other investigations.

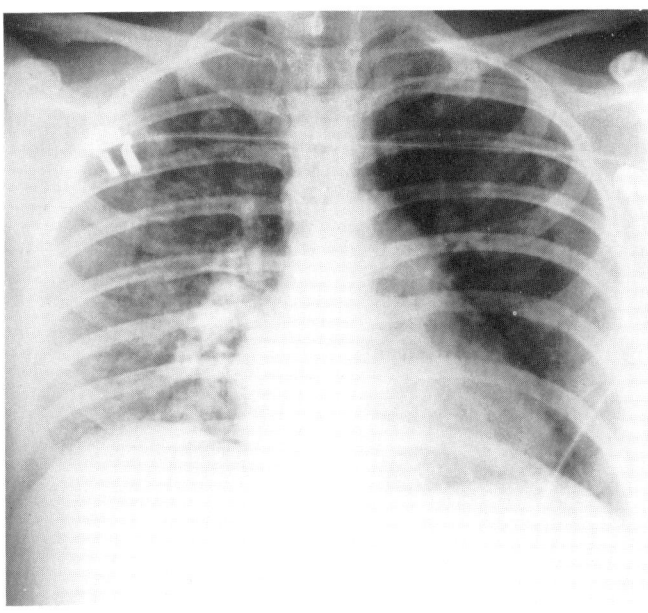

Fig. 10

Answer: Case 5

The heart is normal in size. There are bilateral, diffuse ill-defined opacities in the lung fields. The appearances are those of 'alveolar opacification'. In view of the history of severe trauma fat embolism must be considered.

Other possibilities include the causes of alveolar opacification—transudation, exudation, inhalation and infiltration.

The patient was known to have sustained a fracture of her femur (*Fig.* 11). Fractures of the shaft of the femur have a higher likelihood of causing fat embolism than any other fractures.

Fat embolism occurs because fat from the fractured marrow enters the uncollapsible veins of the bones and is transported to the lungs. The diagnosis can be confirmed by the presence of fat globules in the sputum and urine.

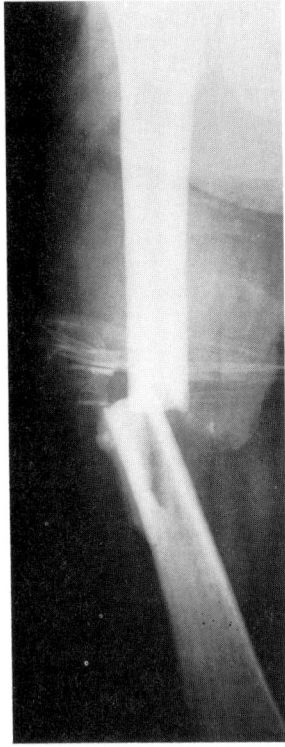

Fig. 11

Case 6

Mrs Andrews, aged 55, was found collapsed in the road. Her supine AP chest X-ray and erect AP films are shown (*Figs*. 12, 13) and lateral films (*Fig*. 14).
Report and suggest further investigations.

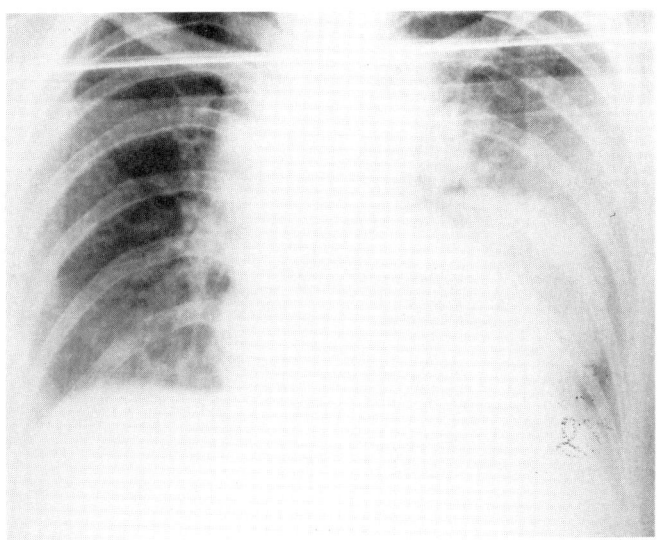

Fig. 12

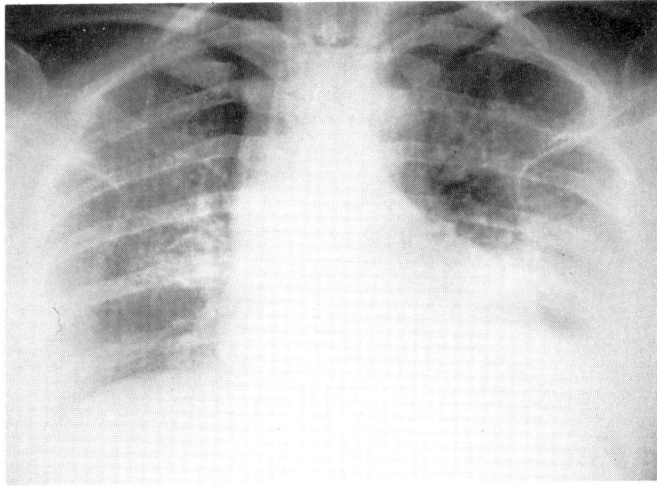

Fig. 13

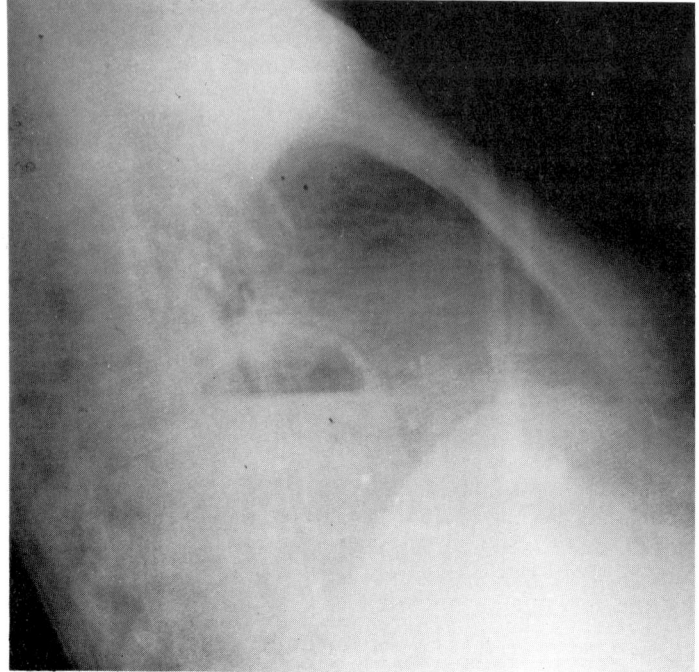

Fig. 14

Answer: Case 6

There is hazy opacification in both lung fields and more confluent opacification in the left lower zone. There is an unusual rounded opacity superimposed on the left heart border on the supine film, widening of the mediastinum and at least two fractured ribs (left 4 and 5).
On the erect films there is a fluid level in the opacity. On the lateral film the fluid level was shown to be posteriorly positioned (*Fig.* 14). The opacity cannot be distinguished from the diaphragm.
Severe chest trauma, consider aortic rupture and diaphragmatic rupture.

Comment

In view of the trauma the mediastinal widening may be due to trauma to the great vessels and angiographic studies for aortic rupture should be considered (*see also* Case 4).
The mass containing a fluid level should alert one to the possibility of rupture of the diaphragm. The condition is of great importance because of the complication of hernial bleeding or strangulation.
Features of diaphragmatic rupture include:

1. Abnormal pattern obscuring the lung base due directly to the herniated bowel. This may give rise to a wrong diagnosis such as subphrenic abscess or traumatic pneumatocoele.
2. Haemothorax or haemopneumothorax.
3. Herniation of the stomach and collapse of left lung may mimic pneumotherax.

Barium studies may be helpful by showing herniation of gut and CT or ultrasound may show herniation of omentum, liver or other viscera

---

Reference

Fataar S. (1979) Diagnosis of diaphragmatic tears. *Br. J. Radiol.* **52,** 375–381.

Case 7

A man, aged 72, had a severe road traffic accident. After some initial improvement over two to three weeks he became more breathless and had increased chest pain. He also became mentally confused. The chest X-ray is shown (*Fig.* 15).

What does it show?

Which other investigations may prove of value in view of the clinical picture?

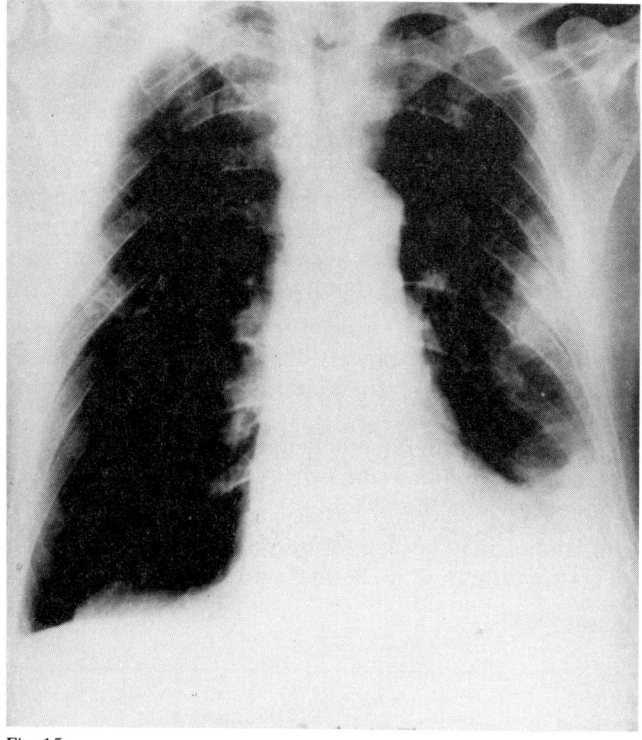

Fig. 15

Case 7

Answer: Case 7

The chest X-ray shows opacification in the mid-zone and at the left base. There are rib fractures of the left 5th, 6th, 7th and 8th ribs adjacent to the opacification. The pulmonary appearances are likely to be due to pulmonary contusion and haemothorax.

In the right hemithorax there is increased radiolucency particularly in the right lower zone. This could be of longstanding (e.g. emphysema) but if comparison with previous films shows that it is a new feature it does raise the possibility of pulmonary embolism.

The next two investigations were a ventilation–perfusion (V/Q) study and CT of the brain (for the mental confusion).

The V/Q scan (*Fig.* 16) shows large defects in perfusion in the right lung but normal ventilation. These appearances have a very high probability of being due to pulmonary embolism. In the left lung there are matching defects corresponding with the contusion.

The CT of the brain (*Fig.* 17) shows bilateral large crescentic areas of low attenuation around the outside of the brain. These appearances are due to bilateral subdural haematomas.

(CT of the Brain is covered in two other books in this series '*CT and MRI Film Viewing*' P. Cook and A. Jones and '*Film Viewing in the Central Nervous System*' by T. Lewis).

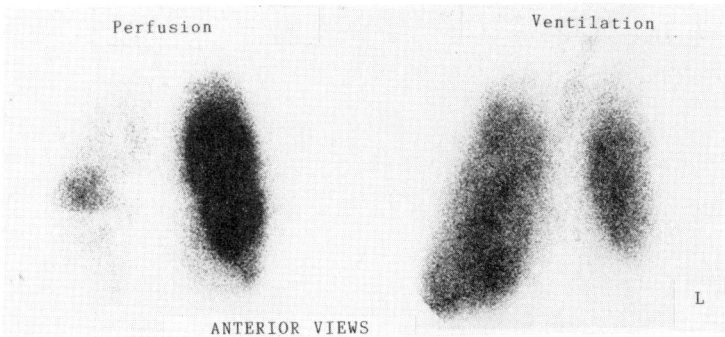

Fig. 16

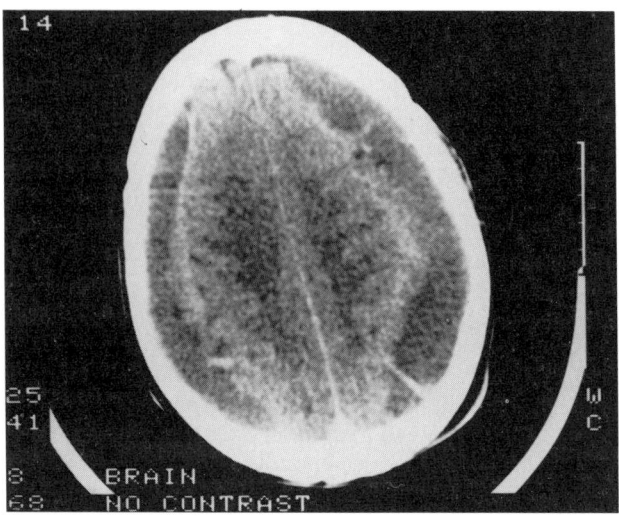

Fig. 17

Case 8

Sue, 25 years of age, has also been involved in a road traffic accident! (*Fig.* 18).

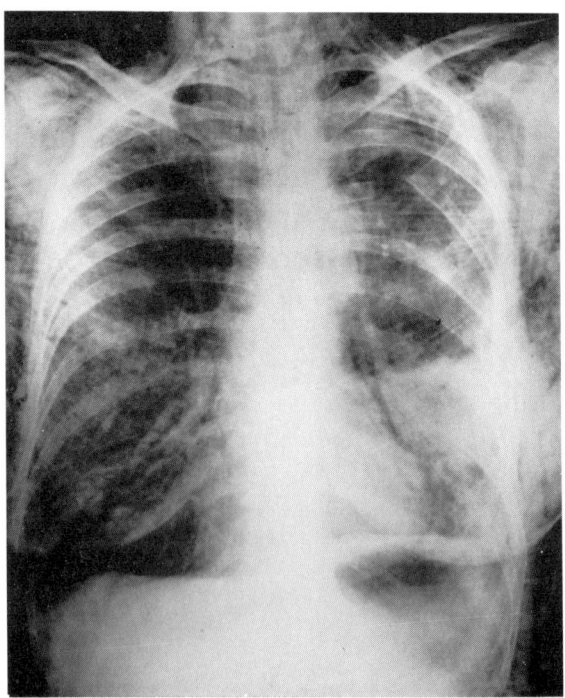

Fig. 18

Answer: Case 8

There is dense opacification in the left lower zone. There is blunting of the left costophrenic angle. There is a fracture of the left 5th rib posteriorly with considerable separation of the fragments.

There are widespread radiolucencies in the soft tissues due to surgical emphysema and there are streaky, linear densities over the lung fields bilaterally due to the air tracking along the pectoralis muscle fibres.

The left *hemidiaphragm* is raised. The pulmonary opacification is due to contusion and haematoma of the lung; blunting of the costophrenic angle is due to haemorrhagic pleural effusion.

The surgical emphysema is the result of air tracking from lacerated lung. The raised hemidiaphragm raises the possibility of diaphragmatic rupture.

(*See also* Case 6)

Case 9

Mavis, aged 30, had a routine chest X-ray (*Fig.* 19).

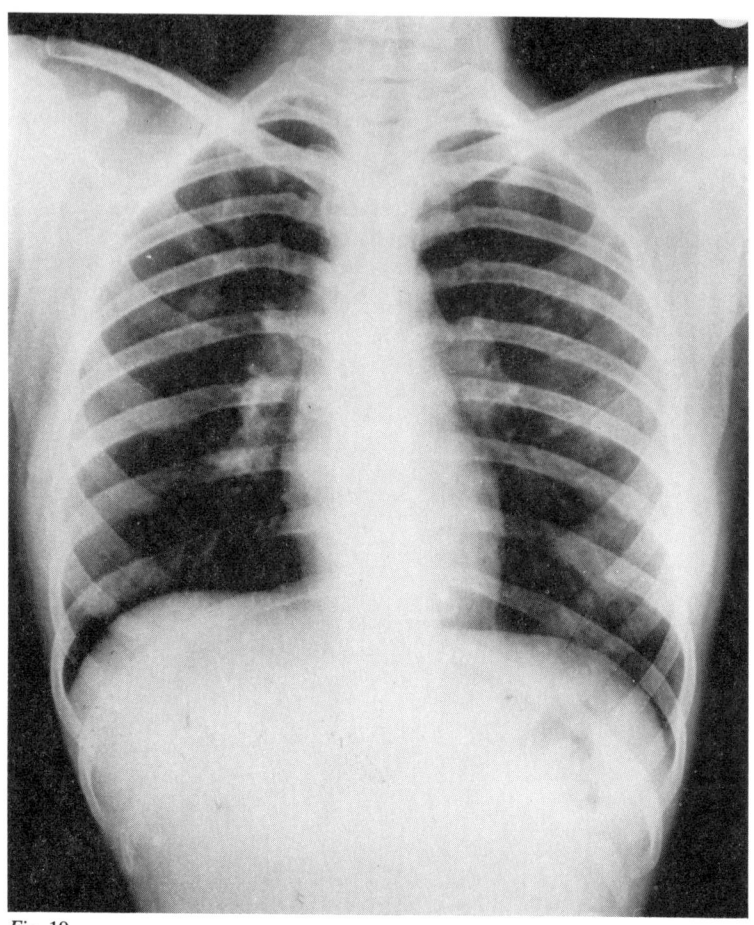

Fig. 19

Case 9

Answer: Case 9

There are ill-defined opacities in both mid-zones. There is enlargement of both hilar shadows with a rather nodular outline. There is slight widening of the mediastinum. The appearances are typical of pulmonary sarcoidosis.

Table 9.1. Causes of hilar enlargement

Common	Bilateral	Unilateral
	Sarcoidosis	Tuberculosis and histoplasmosis
	Lymphoma and leukaemia	Carcinoma of bronchus
	Bilateral pulmonary artery enlargement	Post-stenotic dilatation of main pulmonary artery
		Simulated—mass superimposed on hilum

Less common
1. Pneumoconiosis
2. Viral infection
3. Brucellosis

In suspected sarcoid further investigation can include the Kveim test, biopsy of accessible nodes or of an accessory salivary gland and bronchoscopy and lavage.

Gallium scanning can show a characteristic pattern with increased uptake and enlargement of hilar and mediastinal nodes and uptake in the parotid glands.

Case 10

An adolescent girl, with loss of appetite and a cough, had the following chest X-ray (*Fig.* 20).

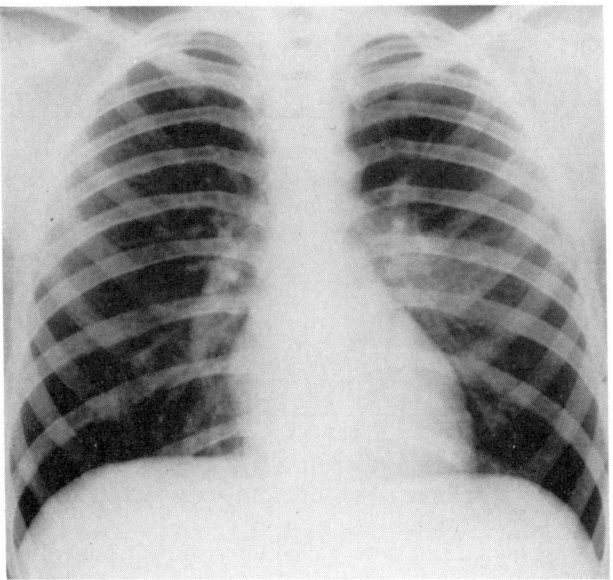

Fig. 20

Answer: Case 10

There is nodular enlargement of the left hilum and adjacent homogeneous opacification. No other abnormality is seen. The unilateral hilar enlargement with pulmonary consolidation is highly suggestive of primary tuberculosis in a patient of this age.

Comment

Primary tuberculosis produces a pneumonia that appears as an area of consolidation. This may occur anywhere in the lungs since, unlike post-primary TB, there is no particular site of predilection. The consolidation is usually single and homogeneous and cavitation is rare.

Enlargement of hilar and mediastinal lymph nodes is common in primary tuberculosis.

In an adult smoker this pattern would nowadays more commonly be due to carcinoma of the bronchus but a young adult or child, TB is still the most important cause with lymphoma being an alternative diagnosis.

Case 11

Vernon, 71 years old, presented with a bloated feeling in his head and neck. His chest X-ray is shown (Fig. 21).

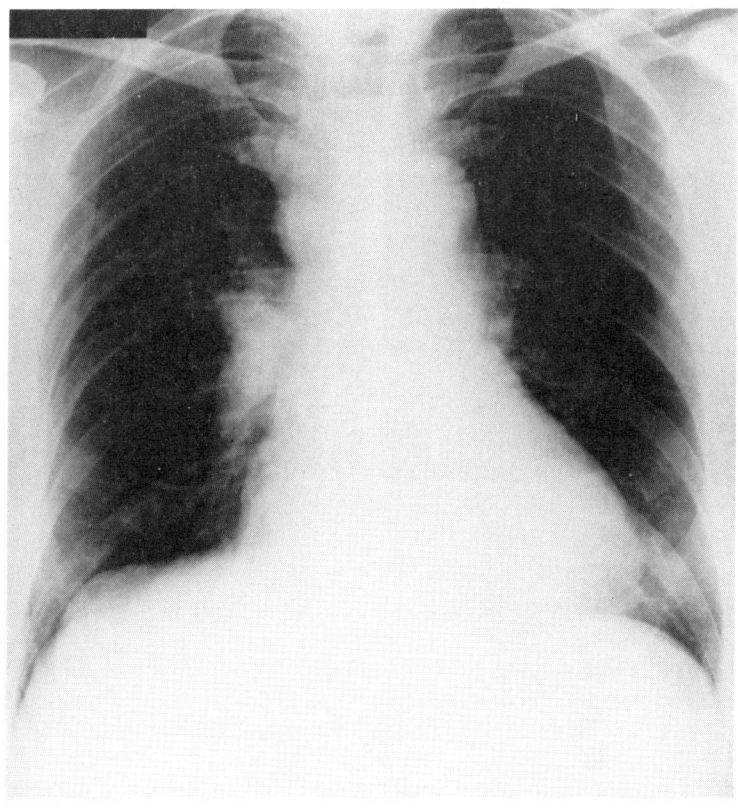

Fig. 21

Answer: Case 11

The heart is slightly enlarged. There is increased density of the right hilum and widening of the mediastinum at the level of the aortic arch and in the superior mediastinum.

A lateral chest X-ray may assist in analysis of the right hilum. The symptoms suggest superior vena cava obstruction (SVCO) and in the presence of a widened mediastinum, computed tomography or venography may be very useful.

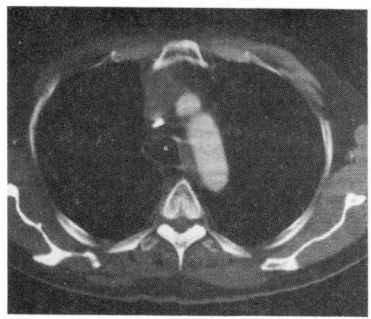

Fig. 22

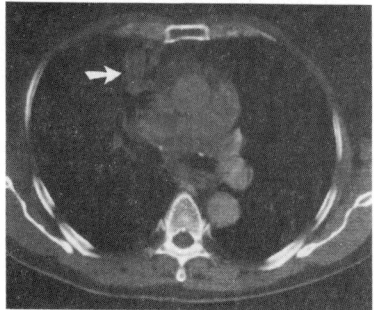

Fig. 23

Further investigation

The lateral chest X-ray (not shown) did suggest the presence of a mass anteriorly.

The CT scans showed a mass anterior to the right hilum (*Fig.* 23 arrowed) and considerable enlargement of lymph nodes in the anterior and superior mediastinum and in the subcarinal region (*Figs.* 22, 23).

Intravenous contrast medium showed the superior vena cava to be obstructed by the lymph node mass.

Conclusion

Carcinoma of the bronchus with mediastinal spread causing SVCO.

Comment

Density of the hilum is an important sign as well as size.

Case 12

The chest X-ray of a young woman (*Fig.* 24).

What abnormality can be seen?

What are the possible causes?

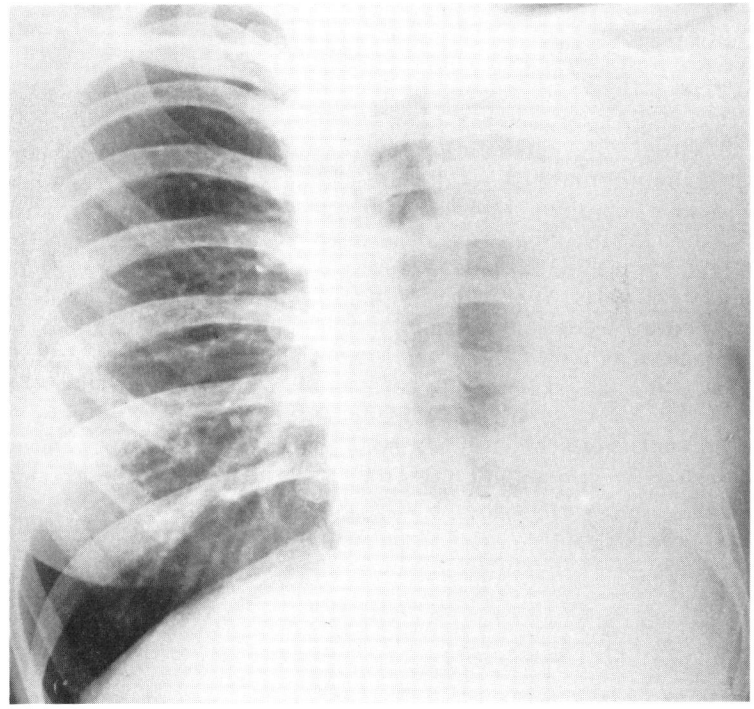

Fig. 24

Answer: Case 12

There is opacification of the majority of the left lung field. The cardiac outline cannot be seen, but there is clearly shift of the mediastinum to the left. There is narrowing of the rib spaces on the left side.

Table 12.1. Opacification of a hemithorax and marked loss of volume

1. Complete collapse or lobar collapse (especially left upper lobe)
2. Hypoplasia
3. Agenesis
4. Pneumonectomy

In this case the patient was known to have agenesis of the left lung. This is a rare condition but it is compatible with life. The hemithorax is smaller than the normal side with narrowing of the rib spaces and elevation of the diaphragm. The heart is shifted into the affected hemithorax and in this case is causing the opacification of the middle and lateral parts of the left hemithorax. The radiolucency in the left hemithorax is due to herniation of right lung across the midline.

Agenesis of one lung is often associated with other congenital defects throughout the body, particularly in the spine, where hemivertebrae are a common accompaniment.

Agenesis must be distinguished from collapse and hypoplasia. This may be difficult and require CT, arteriography or occasionally bronchography. Hypoplasia may go undetected until adulthood and then bronchoscopy may be required to prove that there is no lesion obstructing the bronchi.

Reference

Sutton, D. (1975) *Textbook of Radiology,* 2nd ed. London, Churchill-Livingstone, pp. 449–450.

Case 13

A man, aged 54, presented with loss of weight and a cough (*Fig.* 25).

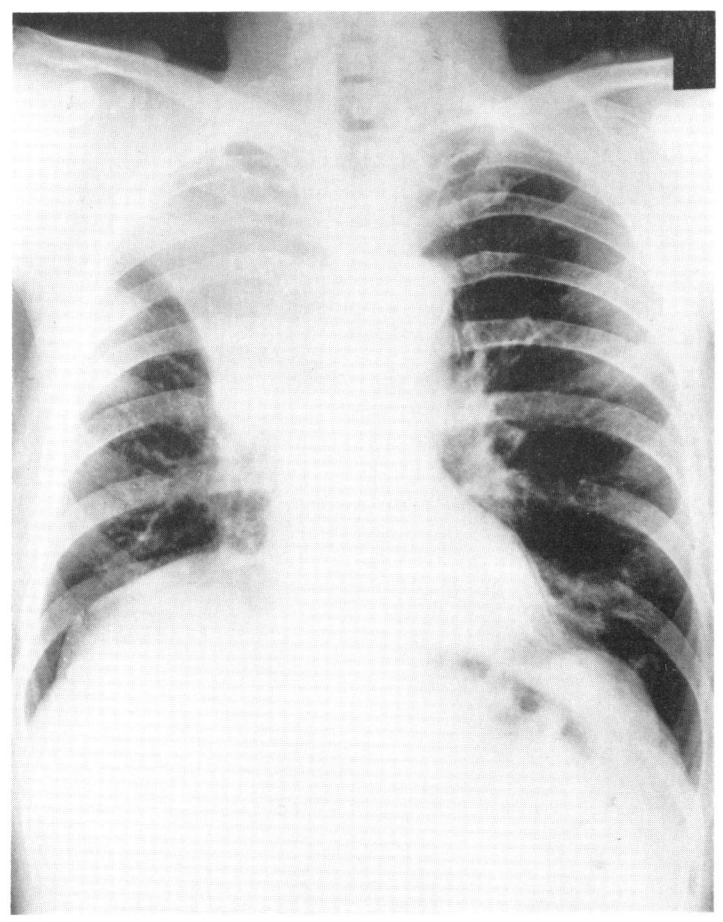

Fig. 25

Answer: Case 13

There is an opacity in the right upper zone merging with the mediastinum. The inferior lateral margin is well defined and extends to the hilum. The right hilum is bulky. The horizontal fissure cannot be identified in its normal site.

In the left lung field there is increased radiolucency. The left proximal pulmonary arteries are large but the peripheral vessels are small.

The right-sided pulmonary opacification is due to right upper lobe collapse associated with a degree of consolidation. The well-defined margin is the displaced horizontal fissure and the bulge at the proximal end, inferiorly, has resulted in a reversed 'S' shape for the outline. This is due to a carcinoma at the hilum obstructing the right upper lobe bronchus. There is emphysema in the left lung.

The patient was a heavy cigarette smoker.

Case 14

A boy, aged 9, presented with exacerbation of asthma. His chest X-rays (PA and lateral) are shown (*Figs.* 26 and 27).

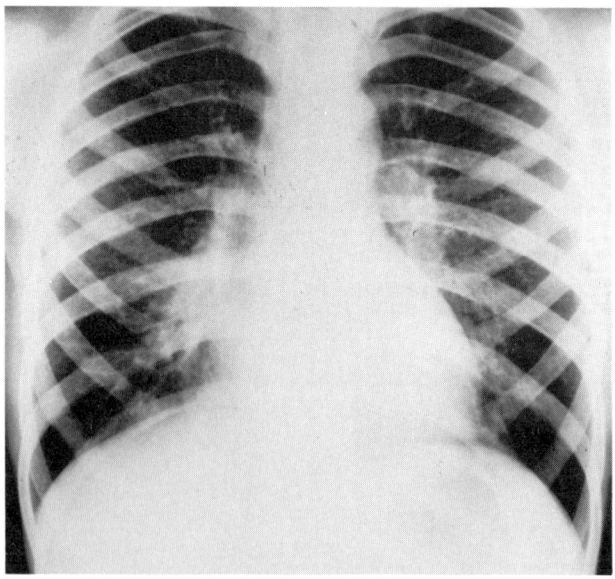

Fig. 26

Case 14

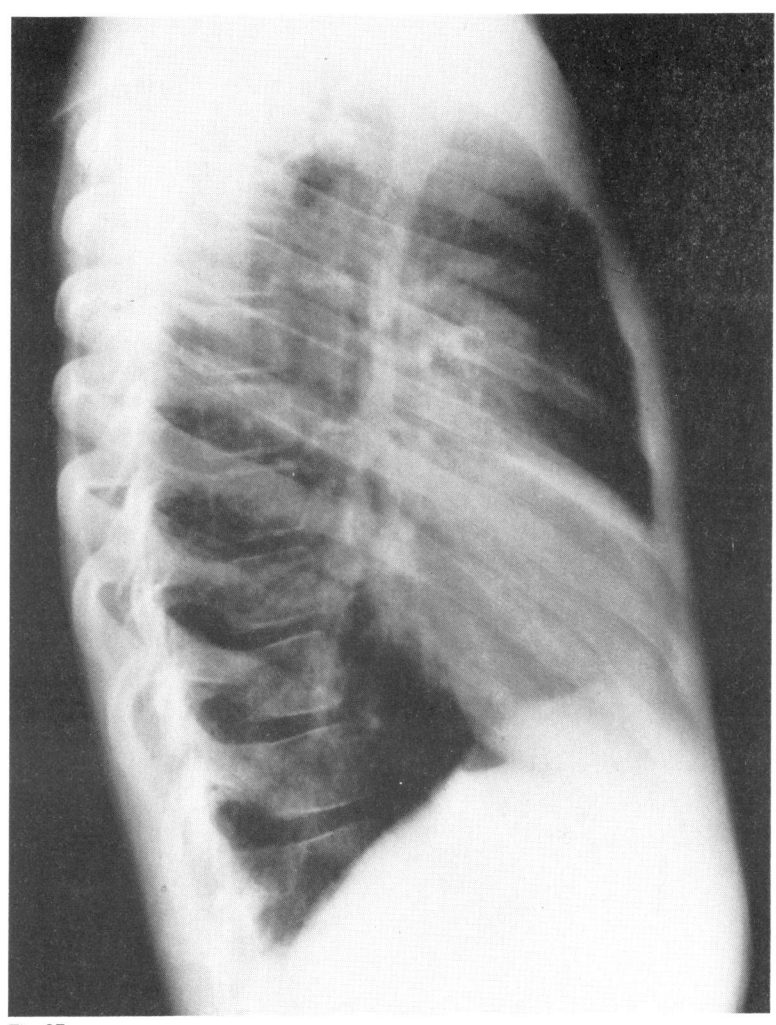

Fig. 27

Answer: Case 14

The right heart border is indistinct. On the lateral film there is a thin white line obliquely in the anterior chest.

The appearances are those of middle lobe collapse. This is due to bronchial obstruction which could be due to lesions in the lumen, in the wall or outside the bronchus.

In this case the collapse was due to 'mucus plugging' due to asthma. Such plugs appear white on macroscopic examination and are interesting in that they are mainly made up of fibrinogen rather than mucus.

The absence of the heart border is an example of an important sign in radiology. The absence of a normal outline implies that there is an opacity abutting the border. In this case the right heart border is lost. This loss of the normal silhouette is known as the 'silhouette sign'.

Case 15

A man, aged 55, presented with haemoptysis. *Fig.* 28 is his PA chest X-ray.

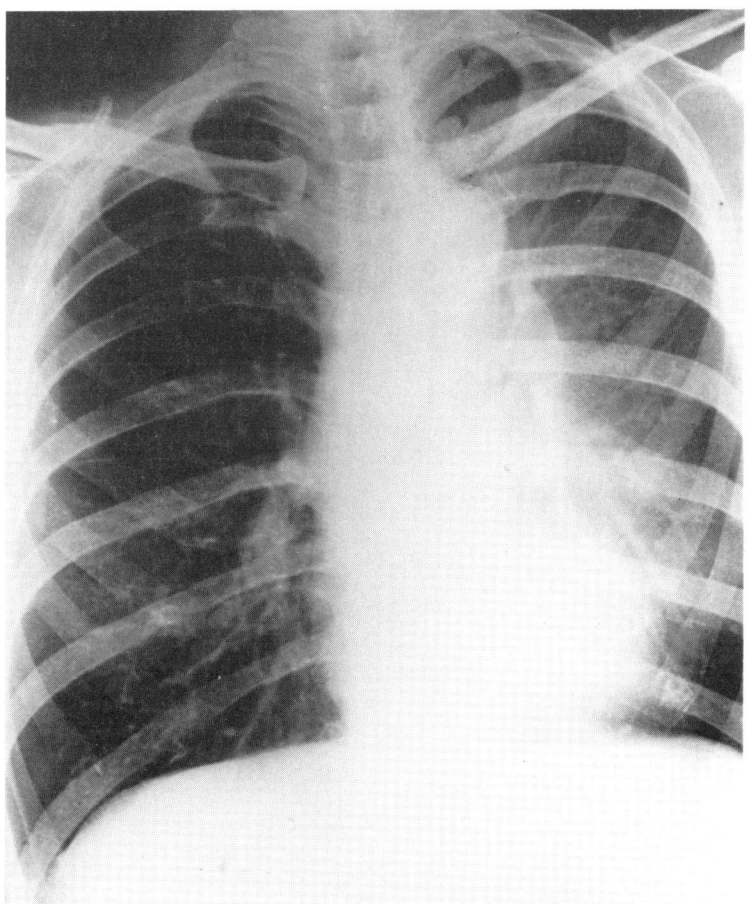

Fig. 28

Answer: Case 15

There is faint homogeneous opacification throughout the left lung field with poor definition of the upper part of the left heart border. The left hilum is elevated and the left hemidiaphragm is slightly higher than the right..

The appearances are due to left upper lobe collapse. The lateral film (*Fig.* 29) shows the collapsed lobe as an opacity anteriorly in the thorax. There is a transradiant area between the front of the opacity and the sternum.

Bronchoscopy was performed and showed a carcinoma occluding the orifice of the left upper lobe bronchus.

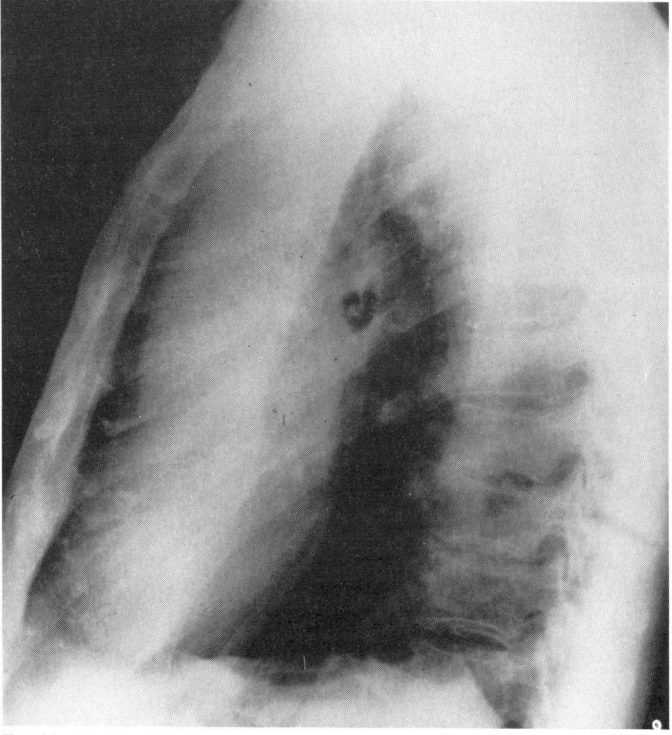

Fig. 29

Case 16

A man, aged 62, with pyrexia (*Fig.* 30).

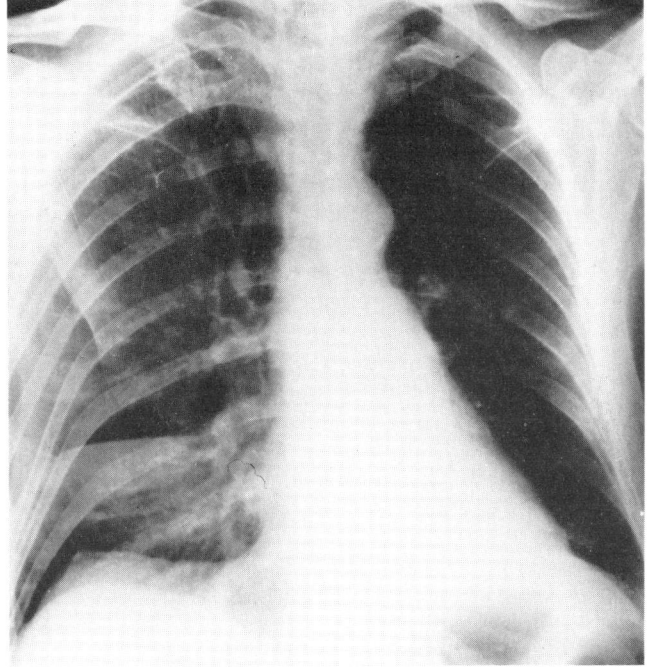

Fig. 30

Answer: Case 16

There is opacification in the right lower zone, the right heart border is obscured ('silhouette sign') but the right hemidiaphragm is clearly shown. The upper border of the opacity is horizontal and clearly defined. There are branching translucencies in the opacity—'air bronchograms'.

The appearances are those of right middle lobe consolidation with upper demarcation due to the horizontal fissure. In the left lung field there is generalized increase in radiolucency. The left hilum is at the same level as the right and there is increased density behind the heart.

These are the appearances of left lower lobe collapse.

Conclusion

Right middle lobe consolidation and left lower lobe collapse.

Comment

The 'silhoutte sign' has been described previously (*see* Case 14). The sign is present where there is loss of an outline due to opacification of adjacent lung. It is thus a sign that assists in determination of the position of an opacity on the plain film.

If there is opacification of alveoli but not of the airways the bronchi will appear as a radiolucent branching pattern against the white background. This is known as an 'air bronchogram' and usually implies consolidation of whatever cause.

The left lower lobe collapse is worrying. If the consolidation and collapse do not respond to antibiotics, bronchoscopy may well be indicated.

A flow chart for the investigation of non-resolving consolidation is shown in *Fig.* 31 and a table of causes of non-resolution of 'consolidation' is shown below.

Table 16.1. Non-resolving consolidation

1. Non-sensitive organism ('wrong' antibiotic)—remember TB and pneumocystis
2. Underlying lung pathology, particularly:
    a. Carcinoma obstructing a bronchus (foreign body in a child)
    b. Bronchiectasis (and bronchopulmonary aspergillosis)
3. Repeated aspiration
4. Immunological deficiency (including AIDS)
5. Non-infective cause of 'consolidation' e.g.
    a. Pulmonary oedema
    b. Pulmonary infarction
    c. Adult respiratory distress syndrome (shock lung)
    d. Contusion
6. Opacity was *not* consolidation e.g.
    a. pulmonary fibrosis
    b. carcinoma of the bronchus
    c. encysted effusion
    (or any other cause of a pulmonary or pleural opacity)

Case 16

Non-Resolving Consolidation

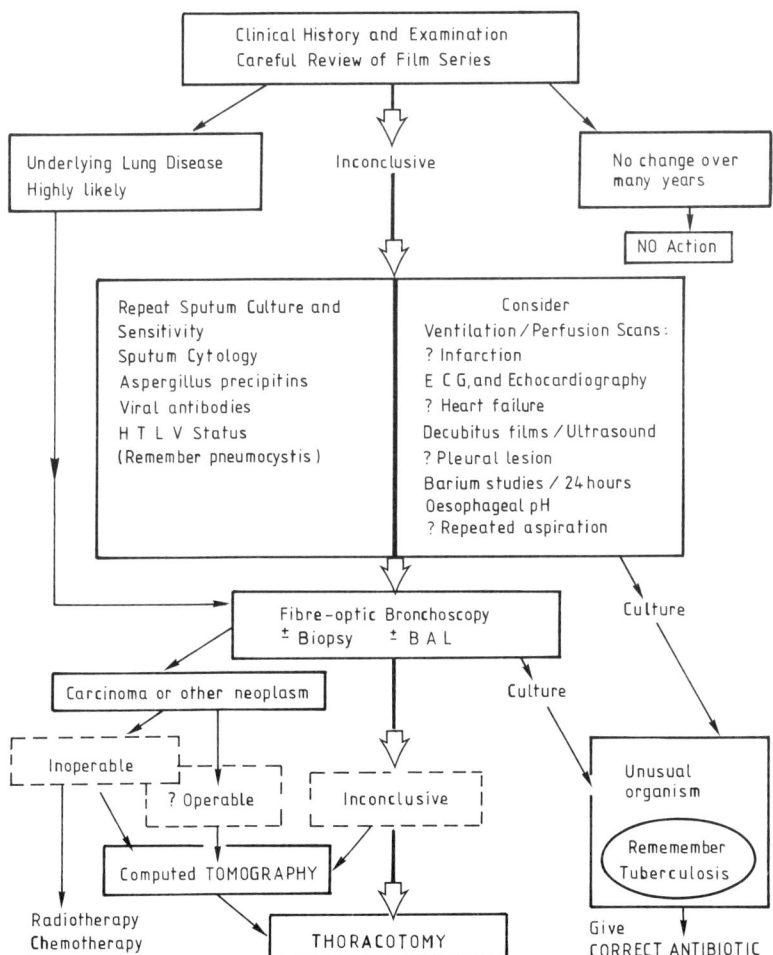

Fig. 31

Case 17

Mr James, 35, had a chest infection which progressed rapidly. *Fig.* 32 is his chest X-ray on presentation and *Fig.* 33 is the X-ray 7 days later.

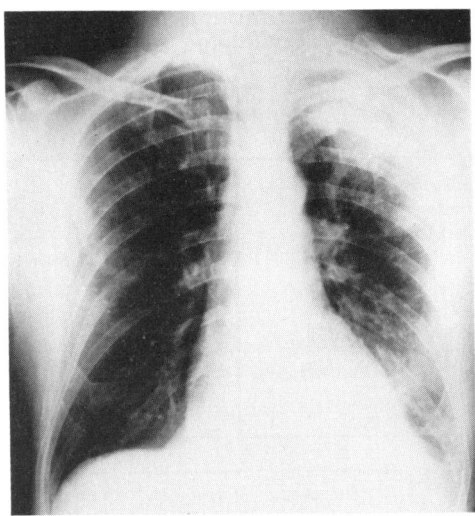

Fig. 32

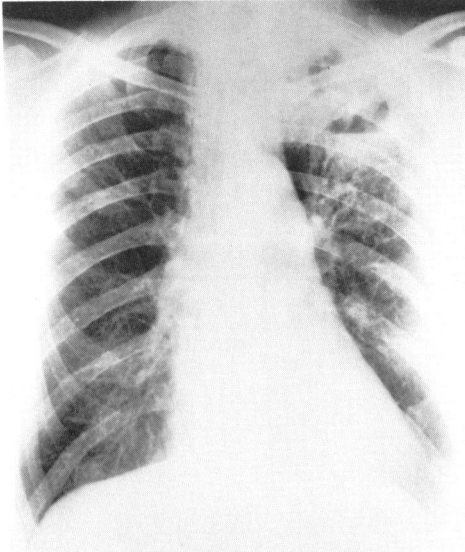

Fig. 33

Answer: Case 17

On the first chest X-ray there is dense opacification in the left upper zone with 'air bronchograms', indicative of consolidation. On the second film the consolidation has broken down into a cavity containing fluid—there is an 'air–fluid level' present.

The most common causes of pulmonary cavitation include carcinoma, tuberculosis, pyogenic infection, trauma and infarction. In the presence of previous consolidation, infection (TB, Klebsiella or staphylococcal) is highly likely. With such rapid progression staphylococcus is likely to be the culprit. This proved to be the case with Mr James.

Unusual or unexpected chest infections in a young adult male should always arouse the suspicion of AIDS (Acquired Immune Deficiency Syndrome). This was not implicated in this case.

Table 17.1. Causes of pumonary cavitation

Common
Carcinoma of the bronchus
Tuberculosis
Pyogenic infection
Trauma
Infarction

Less common
Other malignancies—secondary deposits
　　　　　　　　　　—lymphoma
Sarcoid
Progressive massive fibrosis
Rheumatoid nodule
Cystic fibrosis
Bronchiectasis
Infected bulla
(Mycetoma)—mass within a cavity

Rare
Rare infestations or infection
　histoplasmosis
　coccidioidomycosis
　hydatid

Congenital lesions
　sequestrated segment
　bronchogenic cyst
　cystic adenomatous malformation

Wegener's granulomatosis

Case 18

Pain and weakness in the left arm.
Chest X-ray and CT are shown (*Fig.* 34, 35 and 36).

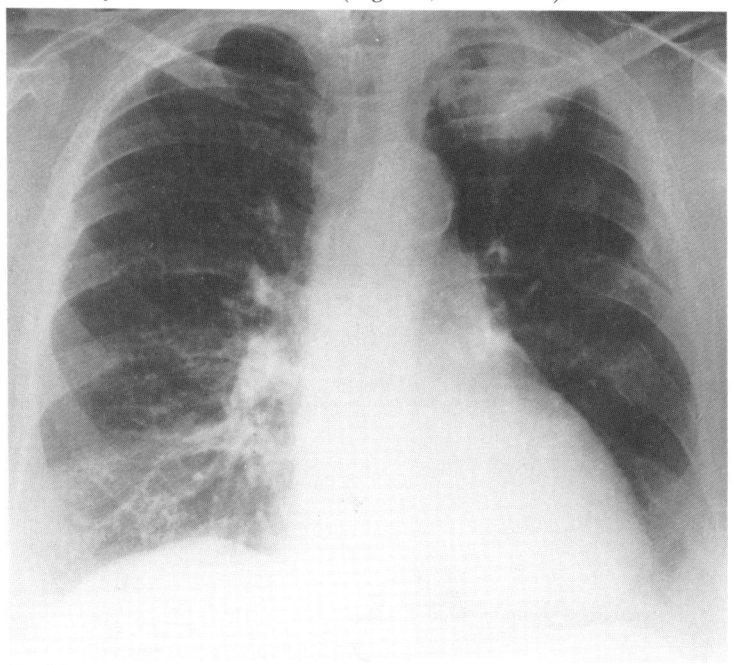

Fig. 34

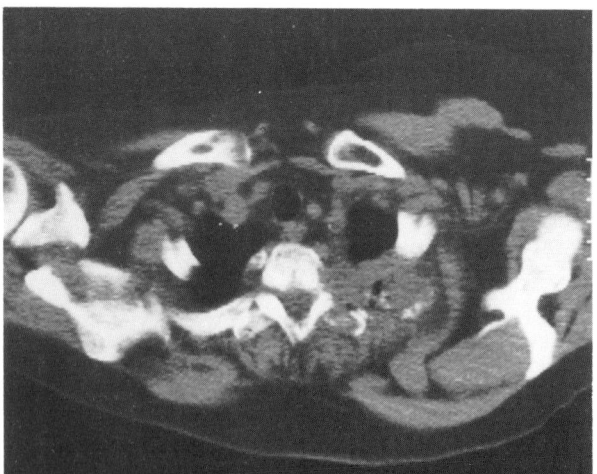

Fig. 35

Case 18

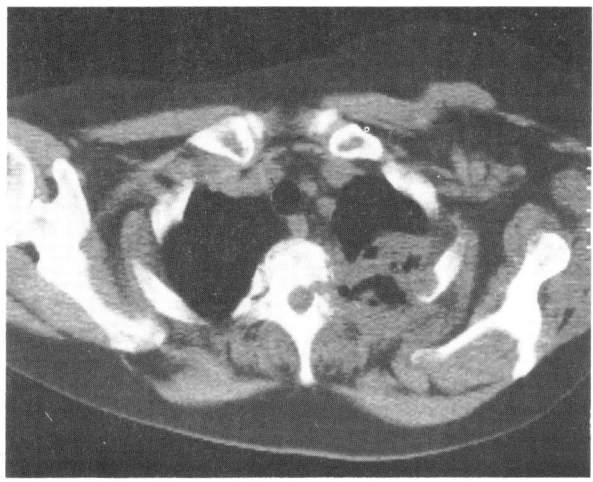

Fig. 36

Answer: Case 18

The chest X-ray showed a mass at the left apex. Old fractures are present bilaterally.

On CT there is a cavitating mass at the left apex. This is seen to be invading the ribs and the pedicle and body of T2.

Conclusion

Cavitating Pancoast tumour.

Case 19

William, aged 50, had a minimal shortness of breath and occasional cough. He also suffered from sinusitis and a skin rash. A chest X-ray and linear tomograms are shown (*Figs*. 37, 38 and 39).

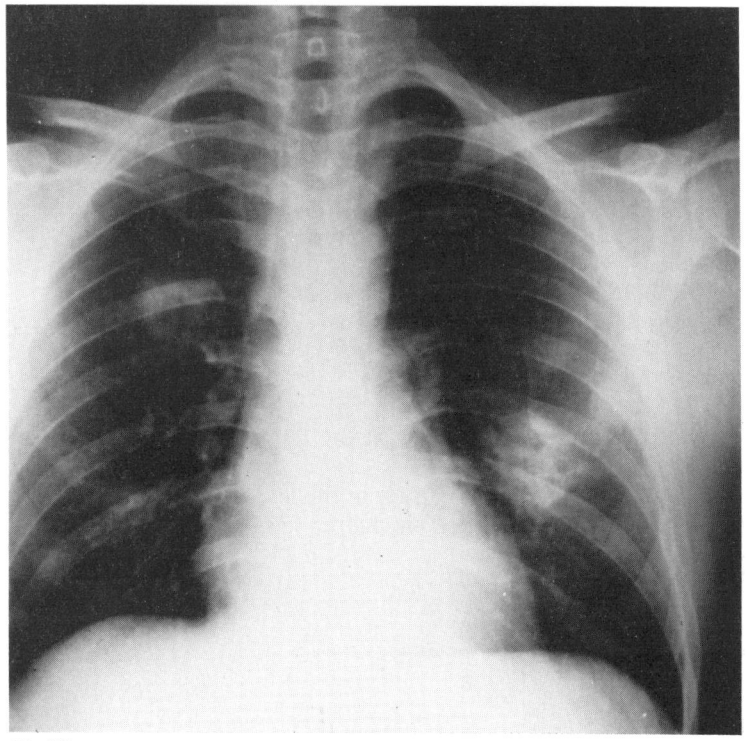

Fig. 37

Case 19

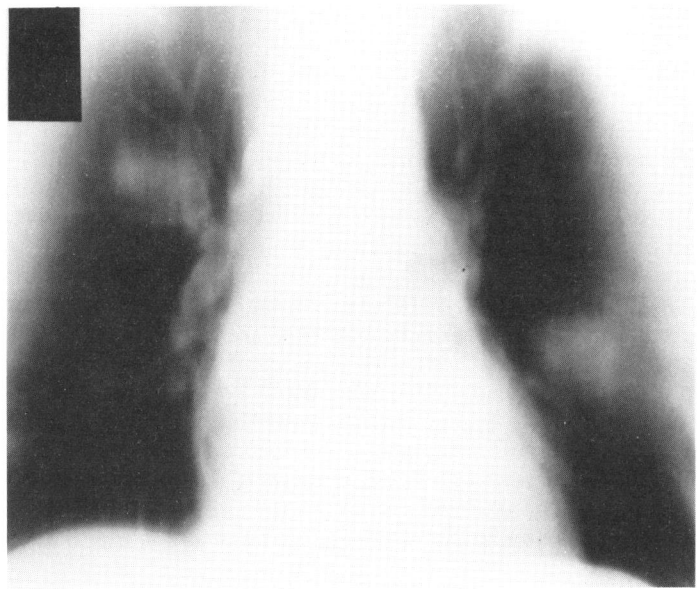

Fig. 38

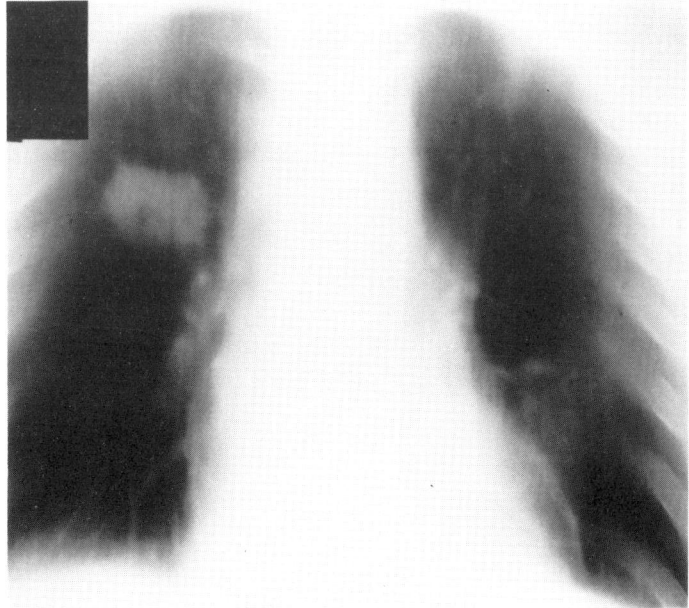

Fig. 39

Answer: Case 19

The chest X-ray shows large ill-defined opacities in the right mid to upper zone and the left mid to lower zone. There are also poorly demonstrated opacities in the right lower zone.

The linear tomography confirms the presence of the right lower zone lesions and shows cavitation in the right upper zone lesions.

Pulmonary cavitation can arise from cavitation in a previously solid lesion or occur as a lesion in otherwise normal lung.

The most important solid mass to cavitate is carcinoma of the brochus. This is usually solitary although pulmonary metastatic deposits from carcinoma of the bronchus are not uncommon.

Multiple metastatic deposits can cavitate. The outlines are usually clearly defined, unlike this case. Poorly-defined cavitating masses can result from infarction, trauma (laceration, contusion and haematoma), abscesses (mainly staphylococcal) and granulomatous conditions (rheumatoid nodules, Wegener's granulomatosis).

The non-pulmonary symptoms were mostly in keeping with Wegener's granulomatosis and this diagnosis was confirmed by histology.

Case 20

Carol, aged 30, had a 3-year history of Hodgkin's lymphoma, treated with chemotherapy and radiotherapy. She was presently suffering from a cough.

Chest X-ray and CT of the chest are shown (*Figs.* 40, 41 and 42).

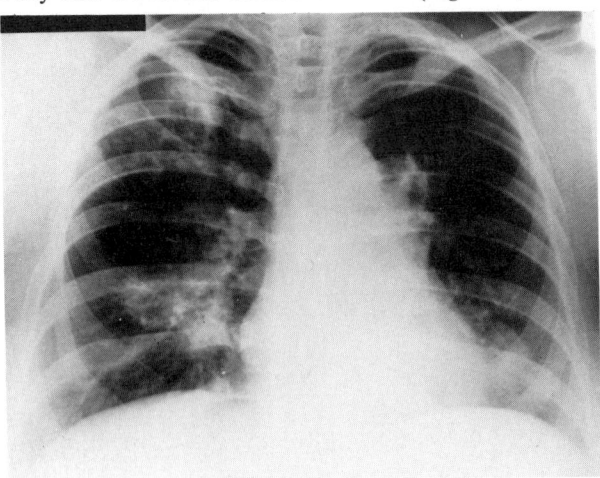

Fig. 40

Case 20

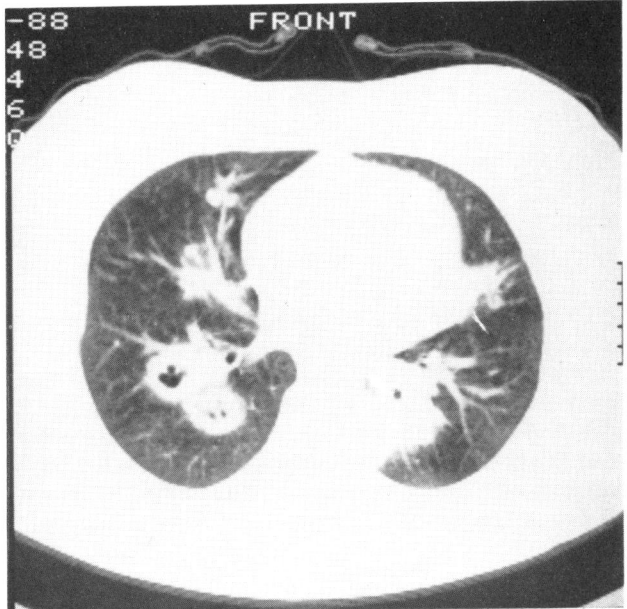

Fig. 41

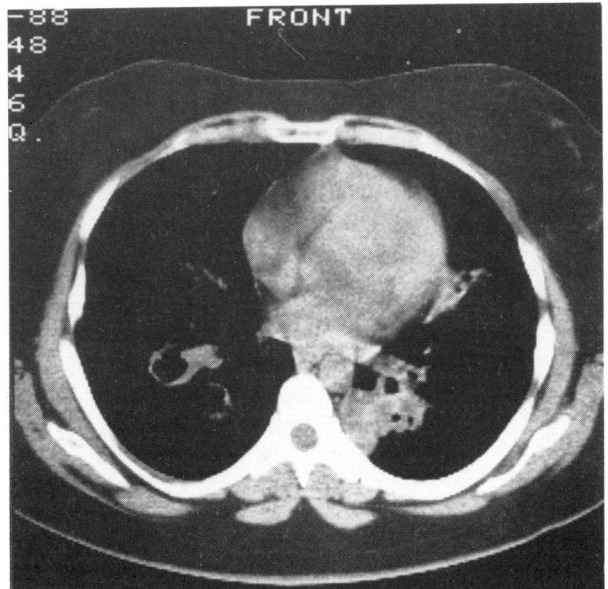

Fig. 42

Answer: Case 20

The chest X-ray shows patchy opacification in both lung fields. There is possible cavitation within the opacities.
 On the chest X-ray findings the possible causes include:
—opportunistic infection
—pneumonitis from chemotherapy or radiotherapy
—recurrence of Hodgkin's lymphoma

Previous chest X-rays showed gradual appearances of the abnormalities.
 The CT confirms the cavitation and shows that the abnormalities are mainly distributed around the outer part of the hila.
 The cavitation would be highly unusual in pneumonitis due to therapy. The unusual distribution is very much in favour of recurrence of Hodgkin's lymphoma rather than opportunistic infection.
 A possible explanation for the distribution is that the mediastinum and main part of the hila have received radiation levels which have prevented recurrence whilst the outer part of the hila were outside the fields.
 Proof of the diagnosis is usually made by histology and open lung biopsy may be necessary.

Case 21

A man with chronic lung disease was noted to have an opacity at the right apex on his latest chest X-ray (*Fig.* 43). The opacity was partially hidden behind the clavicle. It was not present on previous films.
 The lateral film was not helpful with regard to the apical mass. CT was performed (*Fig.* 44).

What do the chest X-ray and CT show?

Case 21

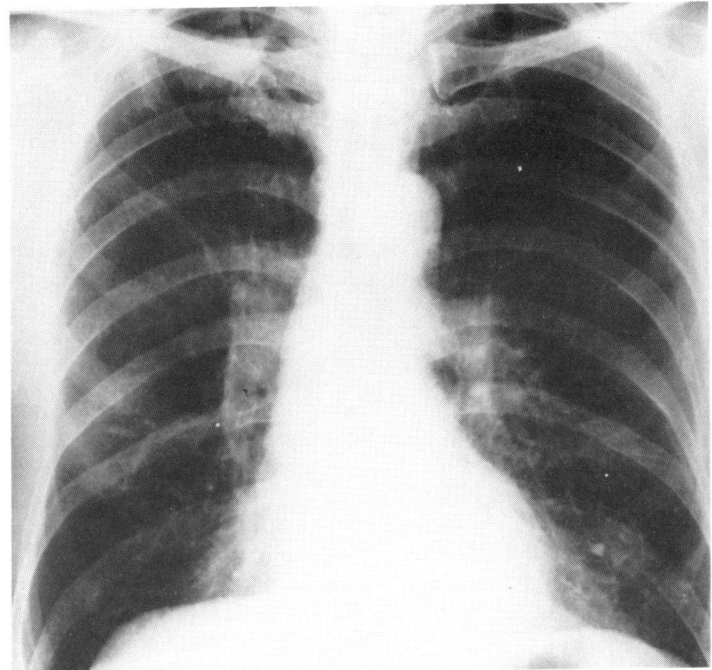

Fig. 43

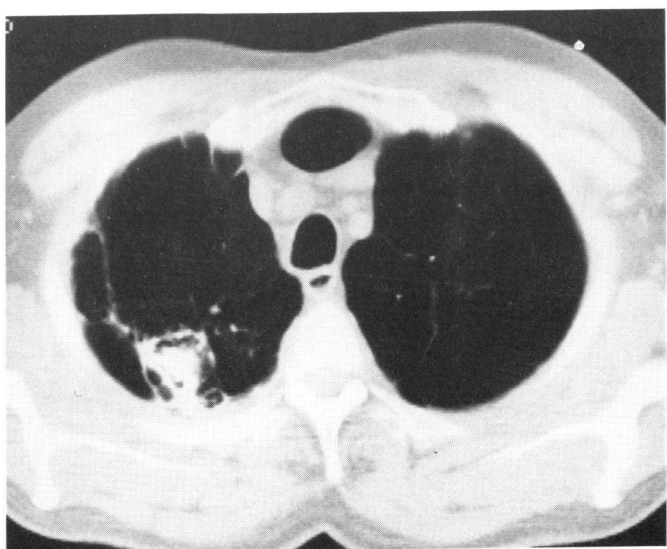

Fig. 44

Answer: Case 21

In addition to the opacity at the right apex the chest X-ray also shows over-expansion of the lung fields and diminished vascularity. A calcified opacity is seen near the left heart border—this represents a calcified TB focus.

The CT shows widespread pulmonary emphysema. The opacity in the right apex is seen to be sited posteriorly. There is an outer dense rim and a crescent of air. The opacity within is only partially solid and contains loculi of air. Mycetoma must be considered and serum tested for aspergillus precipitins.

Comment

In view of the marked emphysema, presumably due to smoking, carcinoma of the bronchus must be suspected. The mass is, however, unusual in configuration for a carcinoma, cavitation in a carcinoma usually occurring centrally rather than around the rim!

The appearances are said to be typical of a *mycetoma* or fungal ball. Perhaps an alternative diagnosis would be a haematoma within a pre-existing cavity. Mycetoma develop in the site of previous lung damage. The fungus will initially adhere to the wall but will separate and develop into a central ball. The main problem is haemoptysis.

Aspergillus fumigatus can affect the lungs in three ways:

1. Mycetoma—fungal ball in a pre-existing cavity, usually from TB or sarcoid.
2. Bronchopulmonary aspergillosis—asthmatic patient with 'autoimmune' response to aspergillus causing bronchiectasis and 'flitting' consolidation.
3. Invasive aspergillus pneumonia—immunosuppressed patient in whom the aspergillus acts as an invasive organism causing a cavitating pneumonia. This is often fatal despite treatment.

Case 22

A sick 16-year-old boy from India (*Fig.* 45).

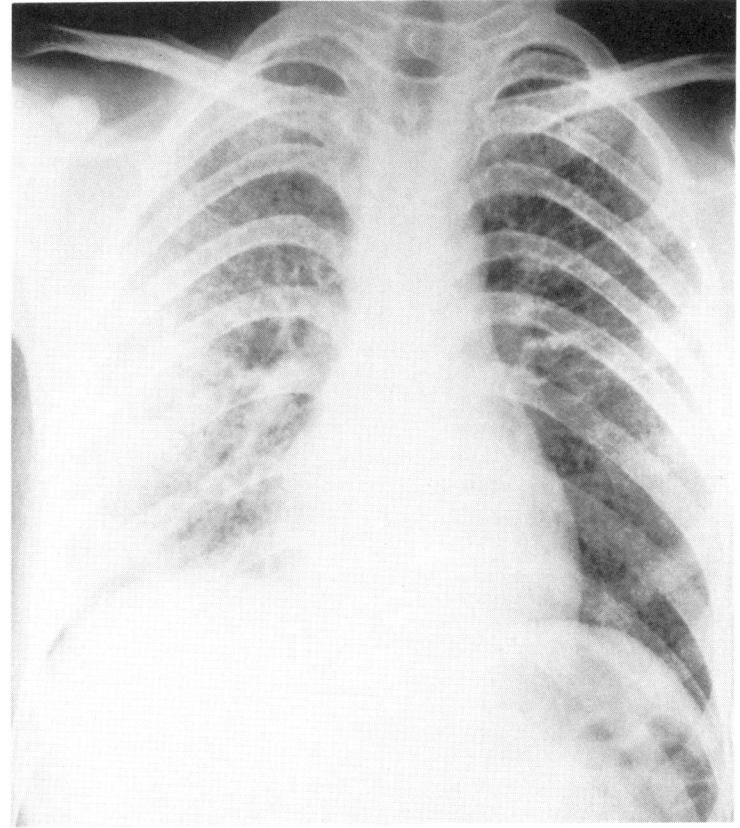

Fig. 45

Answer: Case 22

There are multiple, small, nodular opacities in both lung fields. The nodules are all about 2–3 mm in diameter and are present in all zones with no sparing of the apices or bases. There is confluent opacification in the right lung due to the multiplicity of nodules.

In view of the history and appearances the most likely diagnosis is miliary tuberculosis.

Nodular shadowings are listed in *Table* 22.1.

Table 22.1. Miliary nodularity

Tuberculosis
Sarcoidosis

Cryptogenic fibrosing alveolitis and other fibrosing alveolitides:
   Rheumatoid arthritis
   Scleroderma

Allergic alveolitis
Occupational lung diseases—pneumoconiosis
Metastatic deposits and lymphangitis carcinomatosa

Many other rarer causes including:
   Histiocytosis
   Amyloidosis
   Histoplasmosis and coccidioidomycosis

For causes in childhood see Case 54

Case 23

Mr Davies, aged 58, had a routine employment chest X-ray (*Fig.* 46).

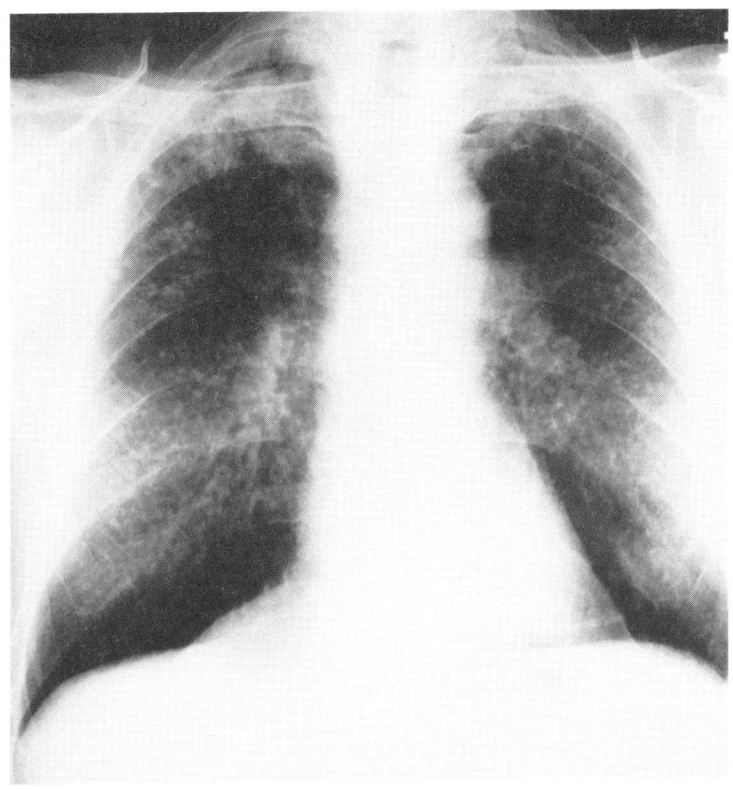

Fig. 46

Answer: Case 23

The heart size and shape are normal. There are multiple 'miliary' nodules throughout both lung fields. In both upper zones there is more confluent opacification.

In view of the lack of clinical symptoms the two most likely diagnoses are pneumoconiosis with progressive massive fibrosis or sarcoid.

Tuberculosis and allergic alveolitis should also be considered. Carcinomatosis and cryptogenic fibrosing alveolitis are the other common causes of miliary nodularity but are unlikely to cause bilateral upper zone opacification. Further investigation should include a very careful history of occupation and hobbies.

Kveim testing, Heaf test and sputum for culture and cytology may be necessary if the history reveals no clues.

In this case long history of coal mining was readily obtained.

Conclusion

Pneumoconiosis with progressive massive fibrosis (PMF).

Case 24

Woman, aged 57, with an irritating cough. Chest PA (*Fig.* 47).

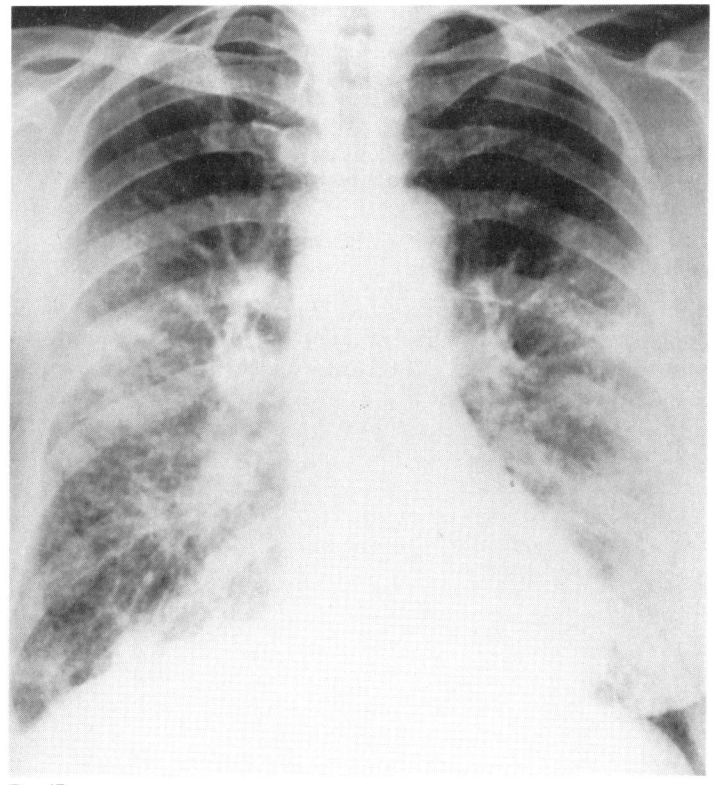

Fig. 47

Answer: Case 24

There is widespread nodular opacification in both lower zones. The close-up of the right lower zone (*Fig* 48) reveals septal lines (Kerley B lines). There are also linear opacities radiating from the hila (Kerley A lines). The heart size is normal. The left breast shadow is clearly seen but the right breast is not seen.

Conclusion
1. Mastectomy for carcinoma of the breast.
2. Lymphangitis carcinomatosa.

Comment
In the presence of a normal-sized heart, septal lines and nodules strongly raise the possibility of lymphangitis carcinomatosa. For examination purposes the mastectomy clinches the diagnosis!

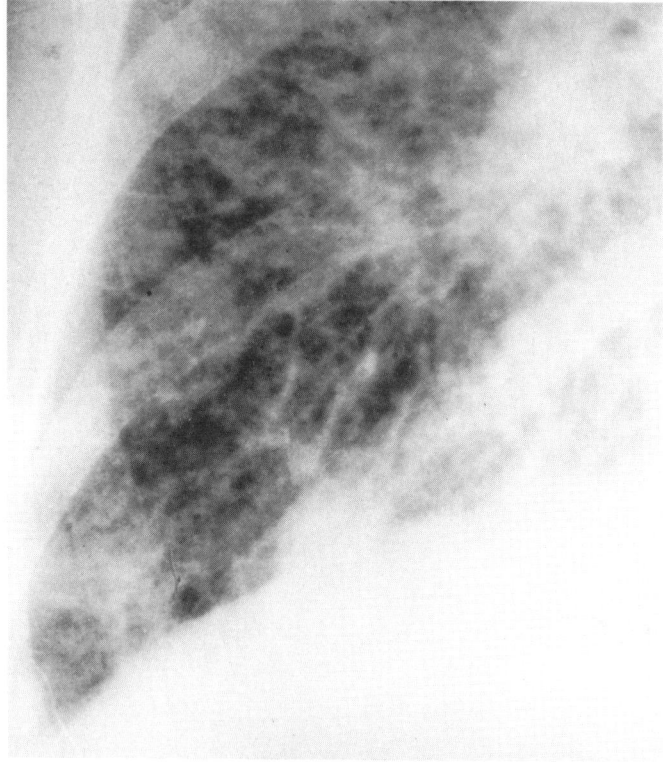

Fig. 48

Case 25

Jack, aged 70, had a productive cough, general loss of energy and dyspnoea. There were scattered râles in the right lower zone (*Fig.* 49).

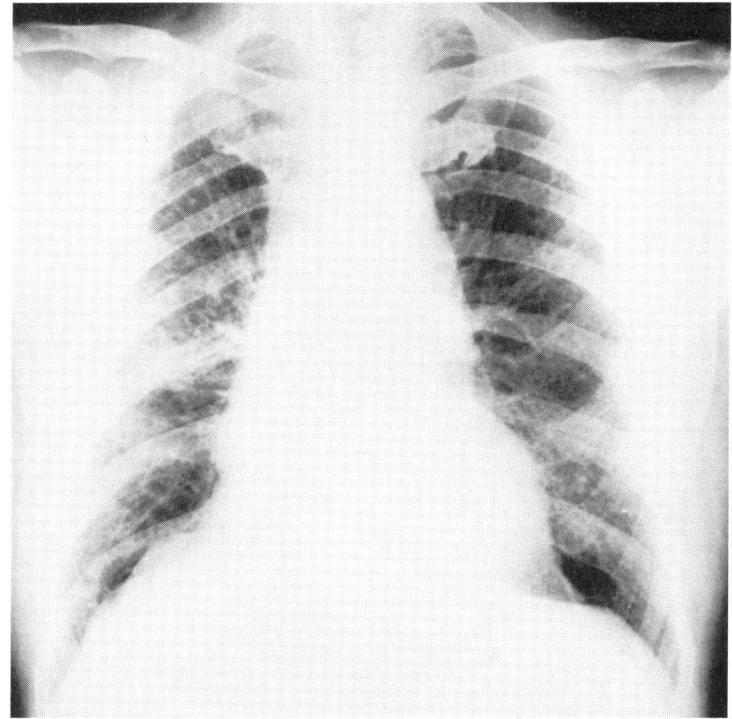

Fig. 49

The chest X-ray showed the heart size to be at the upper limits of normal with associated unfolding of the aorta. There were a few linear opacities in both lower zones. CT of the chest was undertaken to further elucidate the cause of the breathlessness (*Fig.* 50 and 51).

What does the CT show?

What is the likely cause?

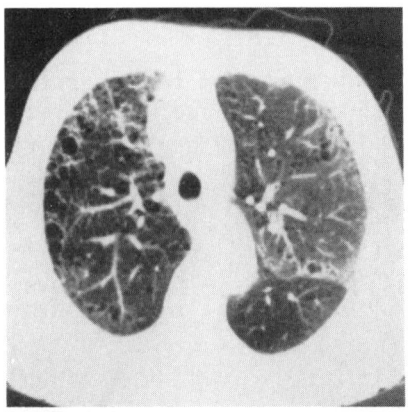

Fig. 50

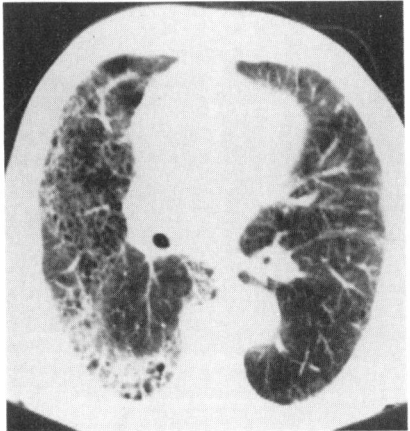

Fig. 51

Answer: Case 25

The CT scan shows small cystic air spaces in both lung fields. These are predominantly peripheral in distribution and are affecting the right lower zone worst of all. The appearances are consistent with fibrosing alveolitis. The same appearances are seen in cryptogenic fibrosing alveolitis and the fibrosing alveolitis associated with connective-tissue disorders such as rheumatoid arthritis and scleroderma.

Similar, but not identical, appearances can be seen in allergic alveolitis, bleomycin lung and asbestosis.

In this case the appearances were considered to be due to cryptogenic fibrosing alveolitis.

Case 26

The chest X-ray of a man aged 50 (*Fig.* 52). This was a well-penetrated film!

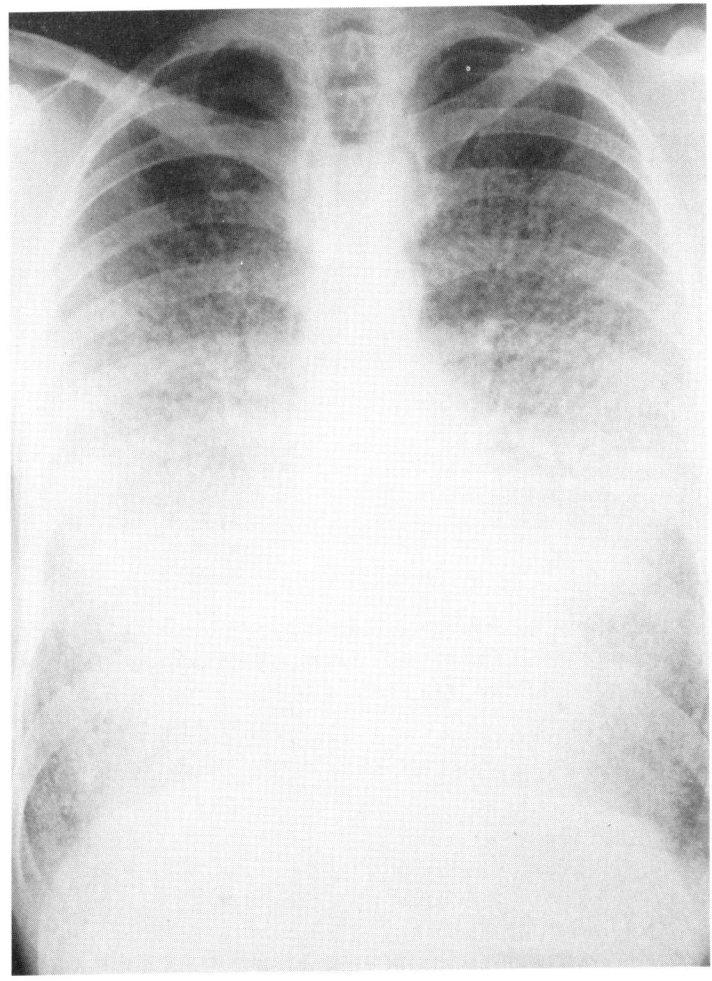

Fig. 52

Answer: Case 26

There are innummerable small opacities of very high density in both lung fields. The opacification is so great in the central part of the mid and lower zones that the heart outline is obscured.
The causes of very high-density, widely-disseminated, small shadows are outlined below (Simon G. (1978) *Principles of Chest X-ray Diagnosis,* 4th ed. London, Butterworths, pp. 108–110.)

Table 26.1. Multiple high-density small nodules

Endogenous
   Haemosiderosis
   Microlithiasis alveolaris
Exogenous
  i. Pneumoconiosis
     Barium
     Calcium (talc)
     Iron (welding, boiler scaling, haematite mining)
     Tin (smelting)
 ii. Post-lymphangiogram
     Oily contrast media
iii. Tuberculosis
 iv. Histoplasmosis
  v. Chicken pox pneumonia
 vi. Ectopic bone (mitral valve disease)

Comment

In this case the appearances were due to microlithiasis alveolaris. In this condition there is endogenous calcification in the alveolar regions of the lung, of unknown aetiology.

Case 27

A chest X-ray from the early 1950s! (*Fig.* 53.)

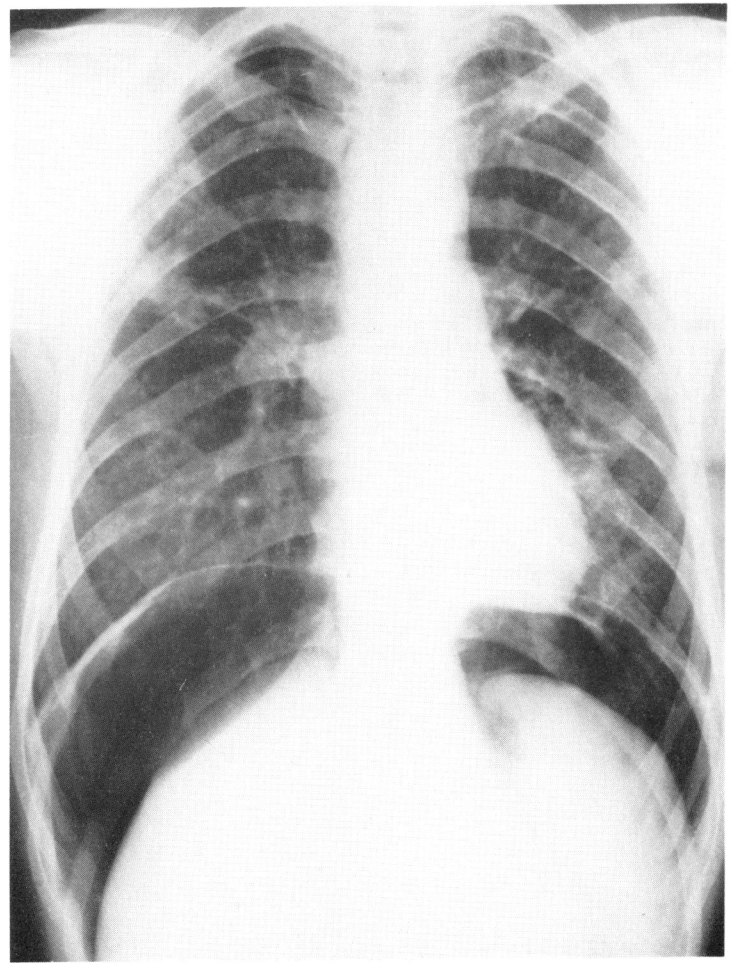

Fig. 53

Answer: Case 27

There is patchy opacification in both mid-zones, the left lower zone and the left apex. There is considerable air beneath the diaphragm within the peritoneal cavity.

The pulmonary opacification is most likely to be due to tuberculosis although bronchopulmonary aspergillosis and sarcoidosis can cause similar appearances.

This patient was suffering from tuberculosis. The pneumoperitoneum had been artificially induced in a similar manner to therapeutic pneumothorax and with the same aim in mind.

Table 27.1. 'Air in the wrong place'

Air in the wrong place can only get there by three methods:
1. From outside —penetrating trauma, surgery, needling
2. From inside —from an air-containing viscus (e.g. gut or bronchus) —trauma, surgery, perforating ulcer or tumour
3. Made there! —gas-forming organisms —necrosis of tissues —water vapour in joints (vacuum sign)

Case 28

A young lady with acute lymphoblastic leukaemia developed an irritating cough and fever. (*Fig.* 54.)

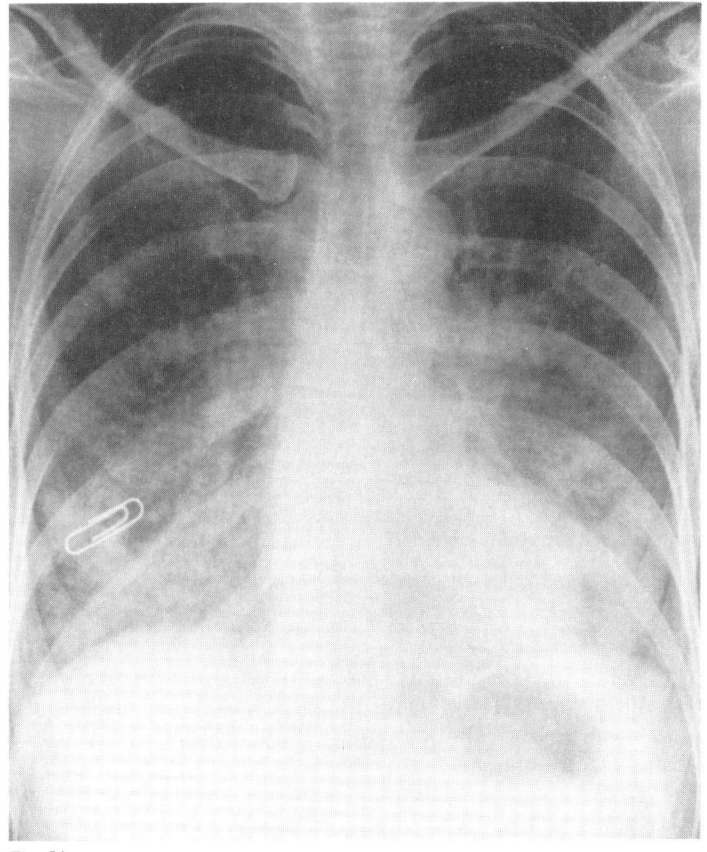

Fig. 54

Answer: Case 28

There is widespread pulmonary opacification with an ill-defined nodular appearance in both mid-zones and confluent opacification with 'air-bronchograms' in the bases.
There is opacification adjacent to the left hilum. The heart size and shape are normal. The pulmonary vasculature is obscured but the upper-zone vessels are visible and are not markedly distended.
The appearances are those of 'alveolar opacification'.
This may be due to a large number of conditions but they can be classified as below.

Table 28.1. Causes of alveolar opacification

1. Transudation (e.g. heart failure, renal failure, overtransfusion)
2. Exudation (infection, proteinosis, haemorrhage)
3. Inhalation (aspiration, toxic gases)
4. Infiltration (leukaemia, lymphoma, alveolar-cell carcinoma)

In an immunosuppressed patient with a fever, opportunistic infection must be considered. The important opportunistic infections include:

Table 28.2. Opportunistic infections

Tuberculosis and atypical mycobacteria
Fungal infection (*Aspergillus fumigatus, Candida albicans*)
Pneumocystis carinii
Viral pneumonias (cytomegalovirus, herpesviruses)

In this case the diagnosis of pneumocystis pneumonia was made from sputum cytology. Diagnosis can be very difficult and may require bronchoscopy and biopsy. Treatment with high-dose Septrin (co-trimoxazole) was successful.

Pneumocystis carinii pneumonia is the presenting condition in 60% of AIDS patients.

In these patients the pneumonia has a 20–30% mortality. Treatment is usually with a high-dose co-trimoxazole which may cause hypersensitivity reactions—nausea, vomiting, anaemia and neutropenia. The alternative, and older, treatment is with parenteral pentamidine which may have even more severe side-effects. Nebulized pentamidine has recently been advocated as a potent antiprotozoal treatment for pneumocystis pneumonia.

Reference
Hospital Doctor Vol. C8, No. 31, Aug. 11/18, p. 28.

Case 29

John B, aged 70, had a history of longstanding asthma, cigarette smoking and recent eosinophilia. He had a chest X-ray which showed a small pulmonary opacity (*Fig.* 55). Sputum cytology was negative. CT was performed (*Fig.* 56 and 57). Needle biopsy was considered.

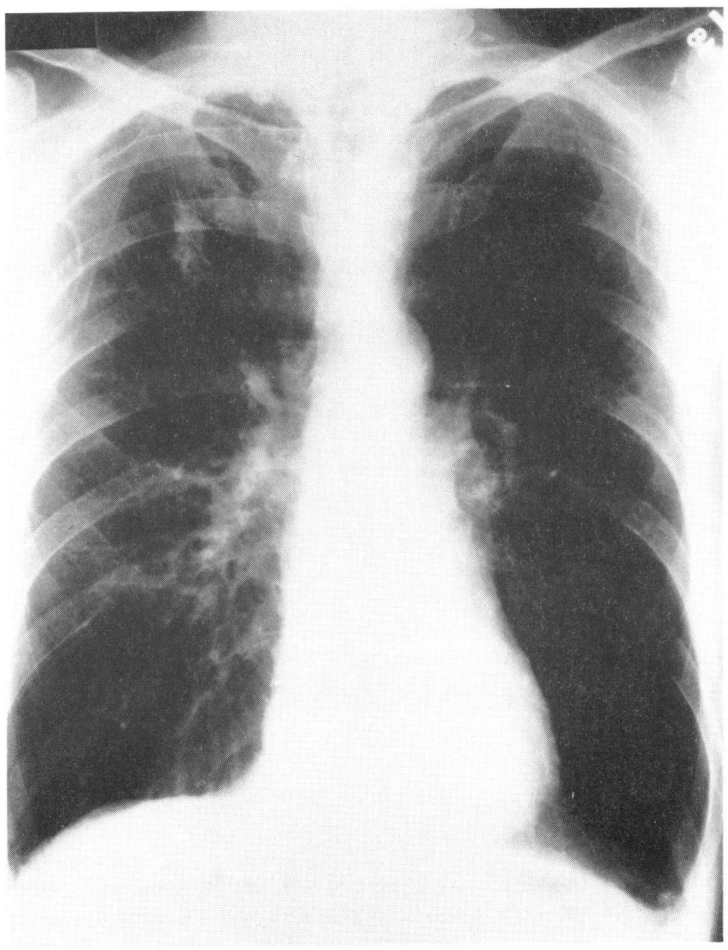

Fig. 55

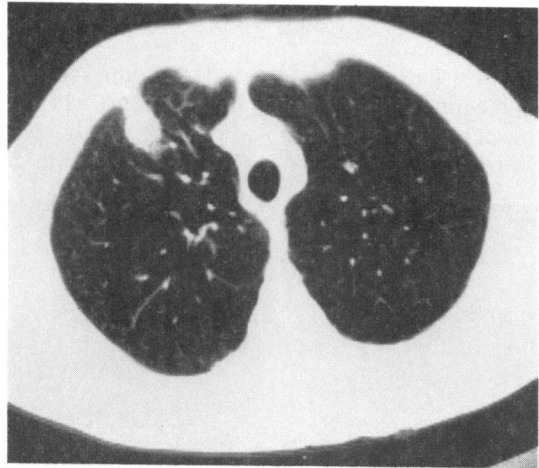

Fig. 56

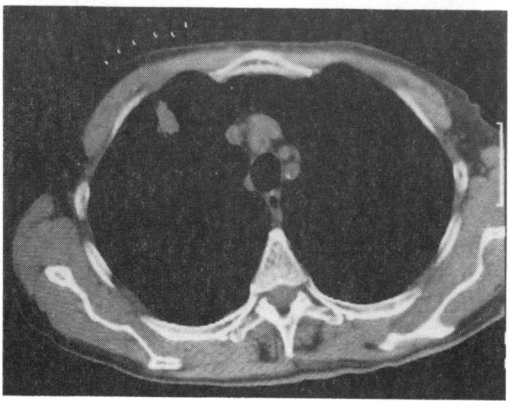

Fig. 57

Answer: Case 29

In addition to the small opacity in the right upper zone there is overexpansion of the lung fields and markedly diminished vascularity. The appearances suggested pulmonary emphysema.

The CT scan clearly demonstrated the lesion which was tethered to the pleura. It also showed pulmonary emphysema of a central pattern. Two diagnoses were considered:
1. Bronchogenic carcinoma
2. Bronchopulmonary aspergillosis

Case 29

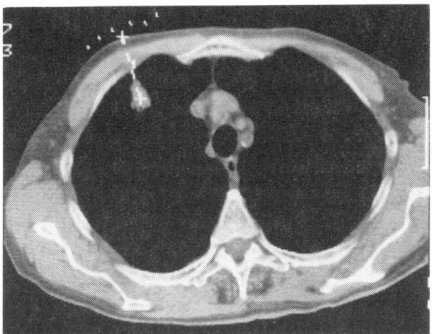

Fig. 58

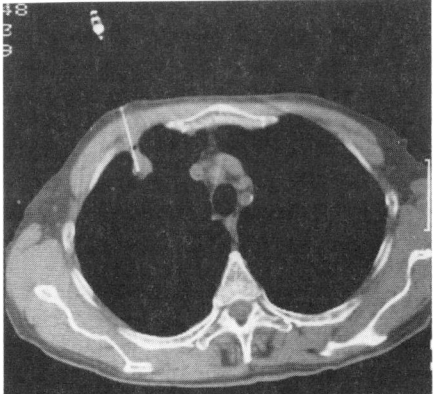

Fig. 59

The latter was considered in view of the longstanding asthma and recent eosinophilia. The history of smoking and the emphysema unfortunately made the diagnosis of carcinoma rather more likely.

The presence of emphysema and the tethering of the mass shown on the CT scan made CT the best method for guidance of the needle biopsy. Fluoroscopy is commonly used for biopsy guidance but it would not be easy to guide the needle specifically through the pleural tethering using fluoroscopy.

Markers were placed on the patient, the needle track and depth were calculated (*Fig.* 58) and the needle biopsy performed (*Fig.* 59). Cytology of the aspirate showed adenocarcinoma.

A flow chart is shown in *Fig.* 60. This should not be followed slavishly and is presented solely as an aid to organized thought about a patient presenting with an opacity on the chest X-ray.

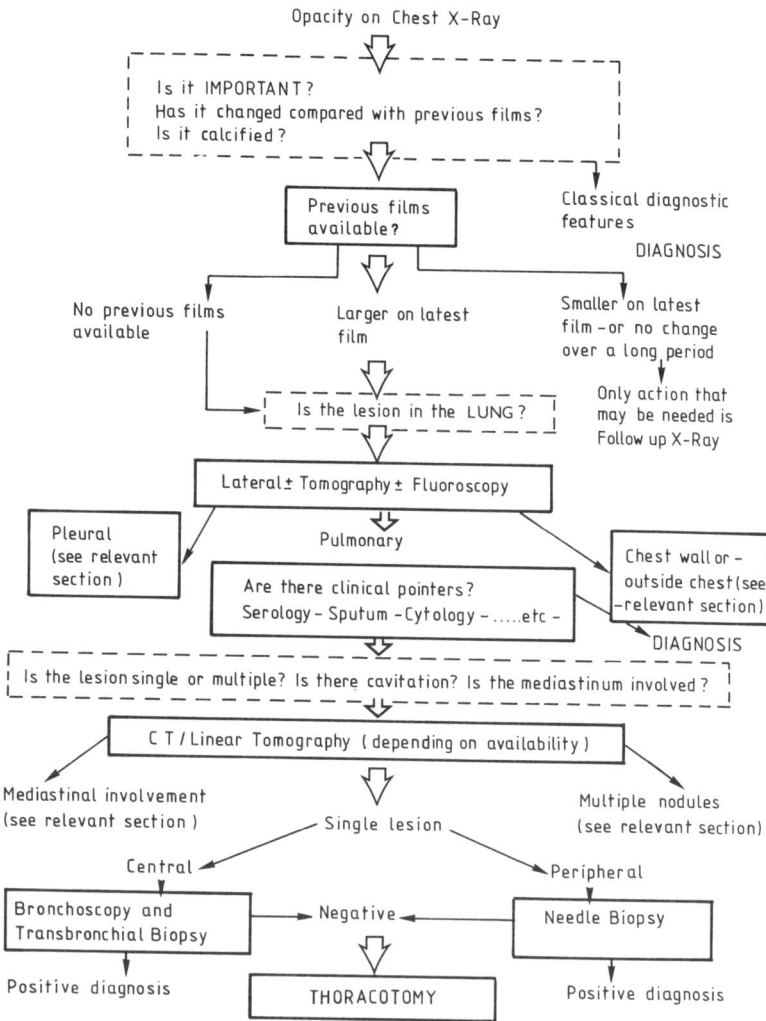

Fig. 60

Case 30

A young Welsh farmer had the following chest X-rays (PA and lateral). (*Figs.* 61 and 62.)

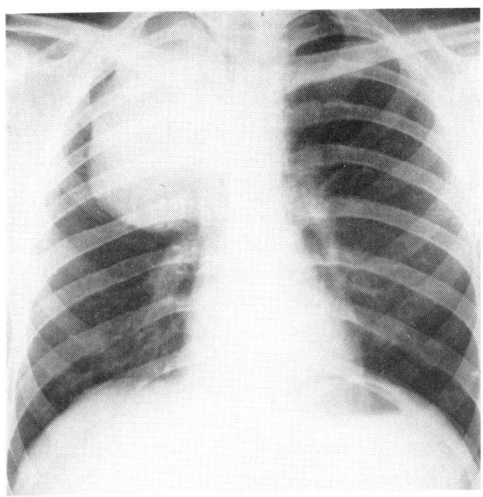

Fig. 61

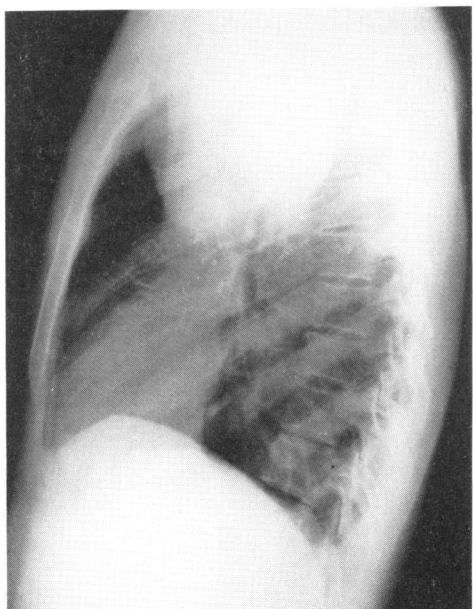

Fig. 62

Answer: Case 30

There is a very well-defined mass in the right upper zone. The mass is dense but no calcification is seen within it. The lateral view confirms the pulmonary location in the upper lobe.

When a large circular homogeneous shadow is seen, and there are no other obvious abnormal pulmonary opacities or bone changes, the list of possibilities is considerable. Frequently there are no clinical clues and further radiology and possible surgery or needle biopsy are required. Calcification may suggest tuberculoma, hamartoma or possibly osteosarcoma deposit. CT may show such calcification and may show other pulmonary lesions such as small satellite lesions. CT may also show abnormal vascular connection, as in an arteriovenous malformation or sequestrated segment, and may be useful in demonstrating that the lesion is cystic rather than solid.

In this case the occupation, sheep farming, the young age and the crisp definition of the edge of the lesion raised clinical suspicion that the lesion was a hydatid cyst. This was confirmed by complement fixation tests.

Hydatid disease is infestation of man with the cystic stage of *Echinococcus granulosus*. The adult worm inhabits the intestines of dogs and sheep are common intermediate hosts.

Table 30.1. Sites of hydatid disease in man

Liver	70%
Lungs	20%
Systemic (kidney, bones etc.)	10%

Case 31

Maria had the following chest X-ray (*Fig.* 63).

What abnormality can be seen?

Could the lesion be malignant?

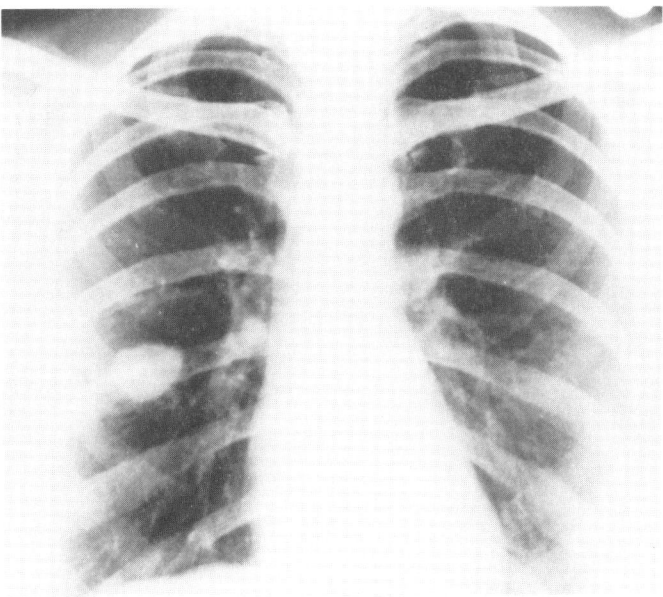

Fig. 63

Answer: Case 31

There is a single well-defined dense opacity in the right mid zone. The opacity is of cacific density. A lateral film would determine whether or not the lesion is intra-pulmonary.

Assuming the lesion to lie in the right lung the possibilities include a massive tuberculous focus (tuberculoma), hamartoma and dermoid.

The only malignant lesions to commonly appear so dense are deposits from osteosarcoma. Such lesions ossify rather than calcify and occur in patients with a known primary osteosarcoma; 'calcification' does not imply a benign diagnosis. Calcification is occasionally seen in carcinoma of the bronchus but is almost never so uniform or so dense as in this patient.

The lesion in this case was a tuberculoma.

Case 32

Mavis (58) had the following chest X-ray (*Fig.* 64).

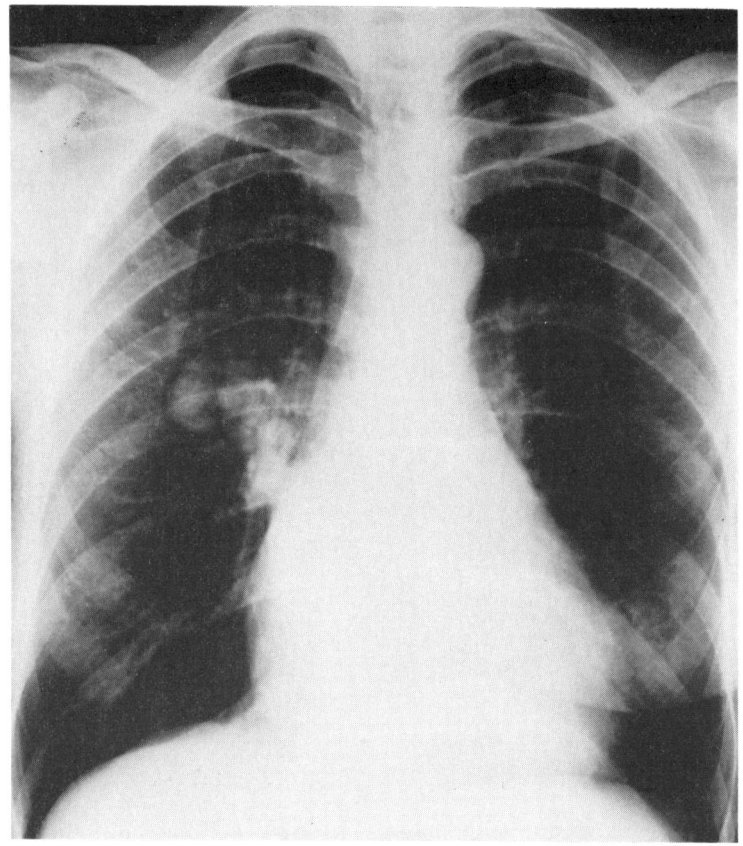

Fig. 64

Case 32

Answer: Case 32

There is a serpiginous opacity adjacent to, and superimposed on the right hilum. No other lung lesion is seen. The heart is slightly enlarged and there is straightening of the left heart border.

The left breast shadow is clearly seen but no right breast outline can be identified.

Conclusion

1. Serpiginous opacity—probably arteriovenous malformation.
2. Mitral valve disease or other cause of left atrial enlargement.
3. Possible right mastectomy.

Comment

On examination both breasts were present but of markedly different size. Always observe the presence or absence of breast shadows and compare with sex—if there is a disparity, a comment should be included in the report, as in this case.

The opacity was confirmed to be an arteriovenous malformation.

Case 33

A female patient, aged 73, with a long history of dyspnoea. (*Fig. 65.*)

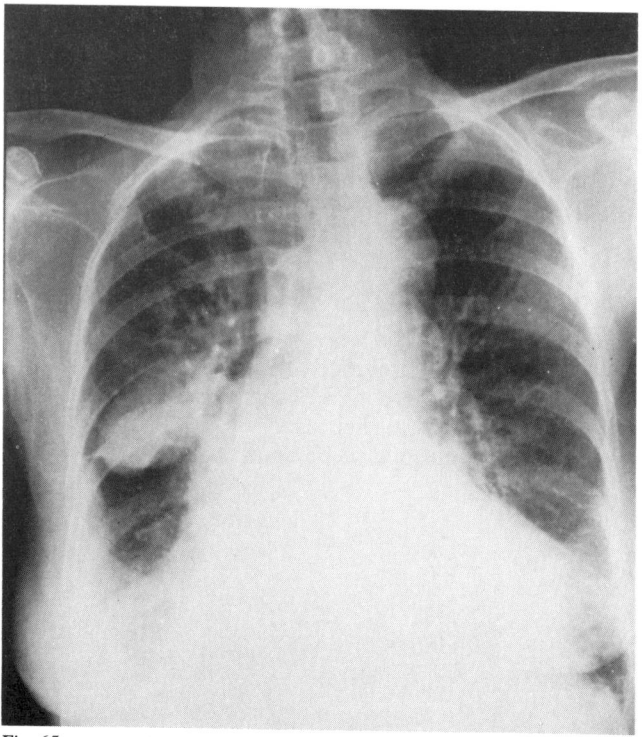

Fig. 65

Answer: Case 33

The heart is enlarged. There is a 'lenticular'-shaped opacity in the right mid zone and blunting of the right costophrenic angle. Septal lines are present in the left lower zone.

The appearances are those of cardiac failure and a right pleural effusion with *encysted effusion* in the horizontal fissure.

Case 34

A man aged 55. (*Fig. 66.*)

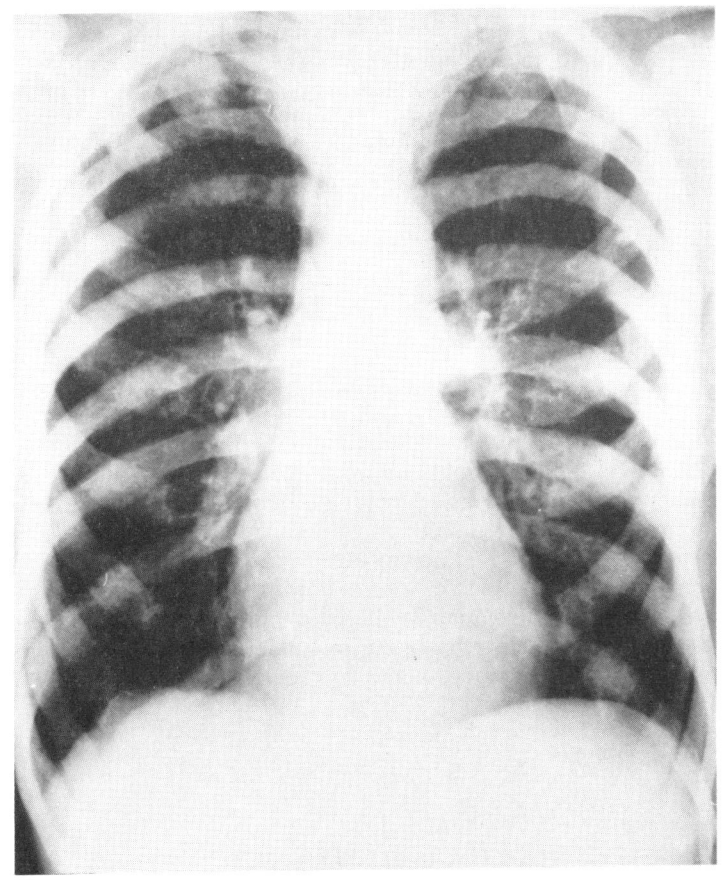

Fig. 66

Answer: Case 34

The major feature is widespread increased density of the ribs. This could be simulated due to a poor exposure. If, however, it is genuine, the most common cause in men is metastatic prostatic carcinoma. There is a small calcific opacity over the left 3rd rib and there is calcification of the left hilum. These appearances are due to old TB.

Table 34.1. Some causes of generalized increase in bone density

Sclerotic metastatic deposits (carcinoma of prostate, breast, lymphoma)
Mast-cell reticulitis (mastocytosis)
Paget's disease
Fibrous dysplasia
Myelosclerosis, myelofibrosis
Fluorosis
Osteopetrosis and pyknodysostosis
Renal osteodystrophy
Sickle cell

In this particular case the patient was known to suffer from oesteopetrosis. This would not have been the first diagnosis to consider without previous history and prostatic secondary deposits were correctly suggested first.

Osteopetrosis, also known as 'marble bone disease' or Albers–Schönberg's disease, affects both sexes and may be familial. There is considerable variability in severity of disease. The bones are brittle and break easily. Osteopetrosis can lead to anaemia, thrombocytopaenia and splenomegaly and leukaemia may develop.

Case 35

Mabel, aged 69, had a productive cough and coarse crepitations in both lungs.

Report on the chest radiograph (*Fig.* 67).

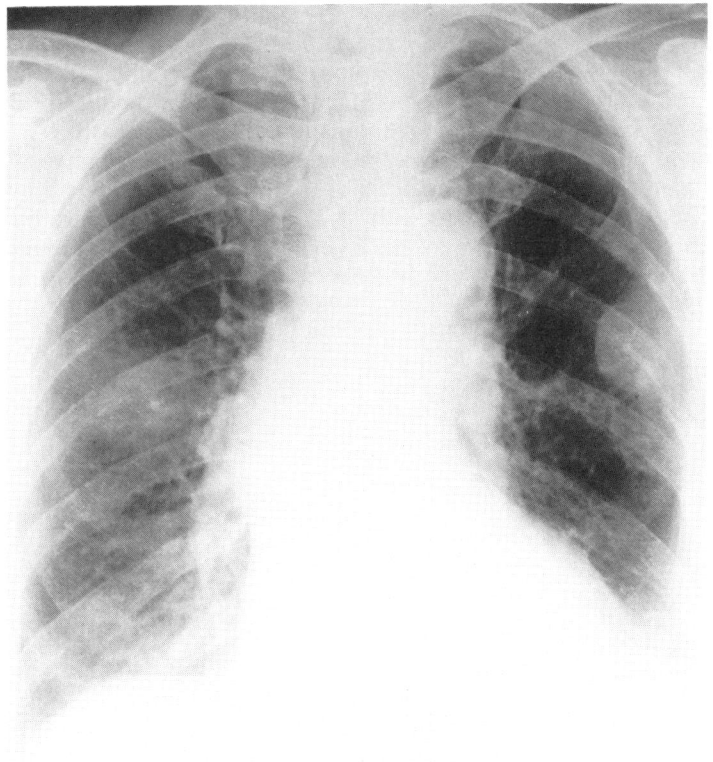

Fig. 67

Answer: Case 35

There is ill-definition of the left heart border and slight pulmonary opacification in the left lower zone.

The heart is normal in size but there is unfolding and widening of the aorta and widening of the superior mediastinum. The latter is likely to represent either a large thyroid or tortuous vessels.

There are opacities peripherally in the left hemithorax with a well-defined medial edge but poorly-defined lateral edge. The *'incomplete border sign'* indicates that the lesions are not contained within the lung but are probably pleural or chest wall abnormalities. Close analysis showed the lesions to be continuous with the ribs. An ill-defined opacity is also seen in the right mid zone. This merges with the anterior end of the right 3rd rib.

The expansile rib lesions with large soft-tissue masses are highly suggestive of multiple myeloma. This condition was confirmed by serum electrophoresis which demonstrated monoclonal gammopathy.

Case 36

Bill, aged 36, presented with systematic hypertension (*Fig.* 68).

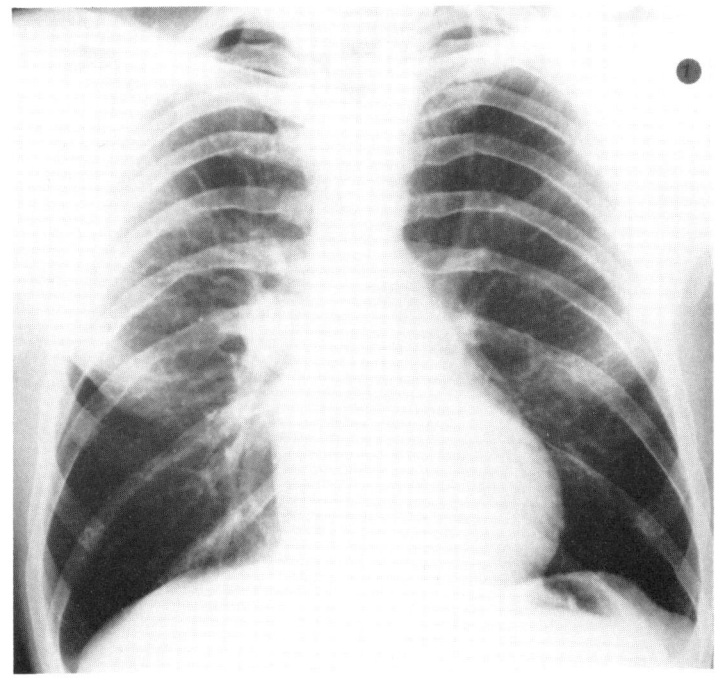

Fig. 68

Answer: Case 36

The heart size is within normal limits. The aortic knuckle is an abnormal shape and there is rib notching affecting the under-surfaces of the ribs bilaterally. The appearances are consistent with coarctation of the aorta.

The cause of rib notching of the under-surfaces of the ribs are related to the structures in the subcostal groove: arteries, veins and nerves. Conditions causing enlargement of these structures are likely to cause rib notching. These conditions are listed in *Table* 36.1.

Table 36.1. Causes of rib notching

Artery	— Collaterals in (a) Coarctation
	(b) Post-Blalock's operation
Vein	— Collaterals in superior vena cava obstruction
Nerve	— Neurofibromatosis

Case 37

Jane had a chest X-ray as part of a 'well-woman' programme (*Figs.* 69, 70).

What abnormality can be seen?

Is the abnormality significant?

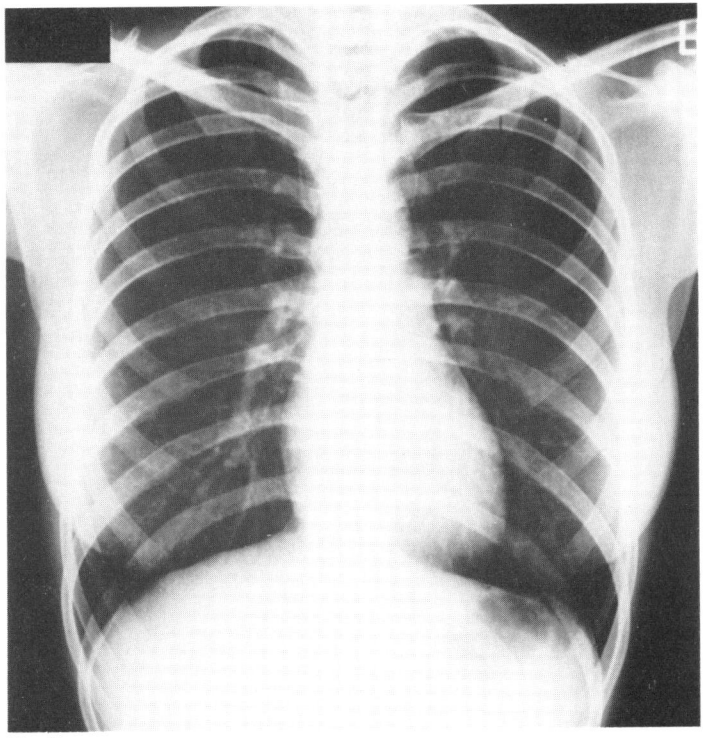

Fig. 69

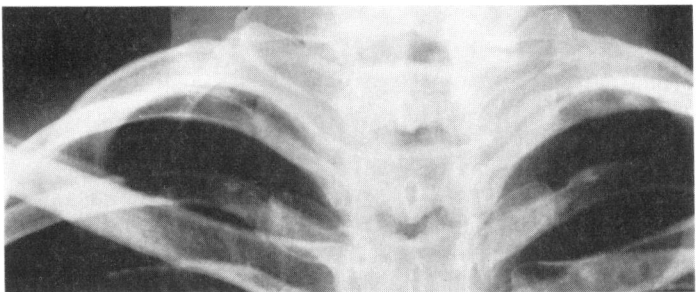

Fig. 70

Answer: Case 37

The heart size and shape are normal. No lung lesion is seen. The only abnormality seen is a small cervical rib on the right side.

This is a common anomaly. Diagnosis is simple, although it may be necessary to count all the ribs in order to distinguish a rudimentary 1st thoracic rib from a cervical rib. Cervical ribs may vary considerably in size. Even a small cervical rib, as in this case, may be significant since it may have a fibrous attachment causing much disability.

Case 38

A woman, aged 35, had a quiet systolic murmur and a cough for one week.

Her chest X-ray is shown (*Fig.* 71).

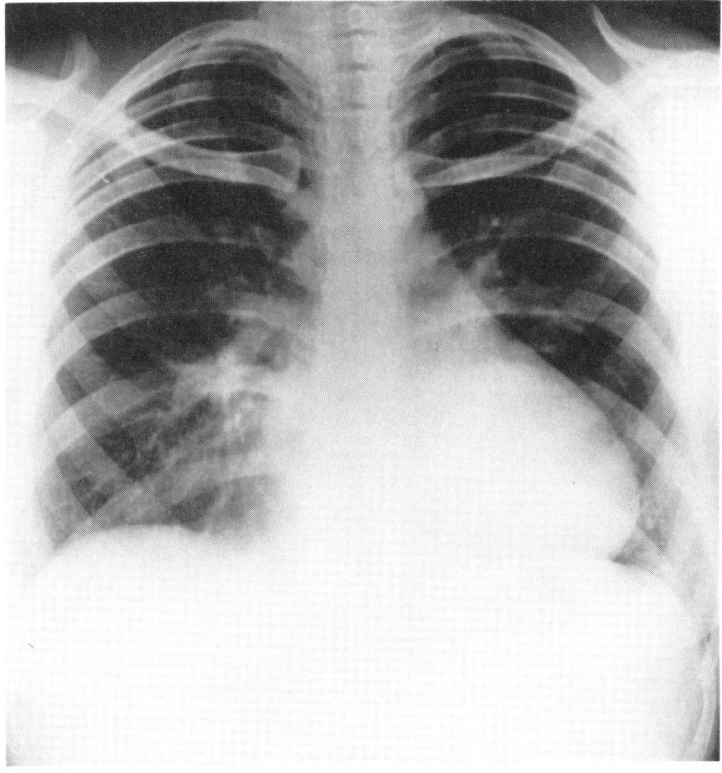

Fig. 71

Answer: Case 38

There is ill-definition of the right heart border. The heart size is at the upper limits of normal in transverse diameter (normal is below 0.5).

The anterior aspects of the ribs are shown to be more vertical than usual, whilst the posterior aspects are horizontal. The appearances are due to 'pectus excavatum' or depression of the sternum.

This is confirmed on the lateral film (*Fig.* 72).

Pectus excavatum is a normal variant in which the sternum may be considerably shifted posteriorly. this may be associated with a mild sytolic ejection murmur and is very occasionally associated with an atrial septal defect.

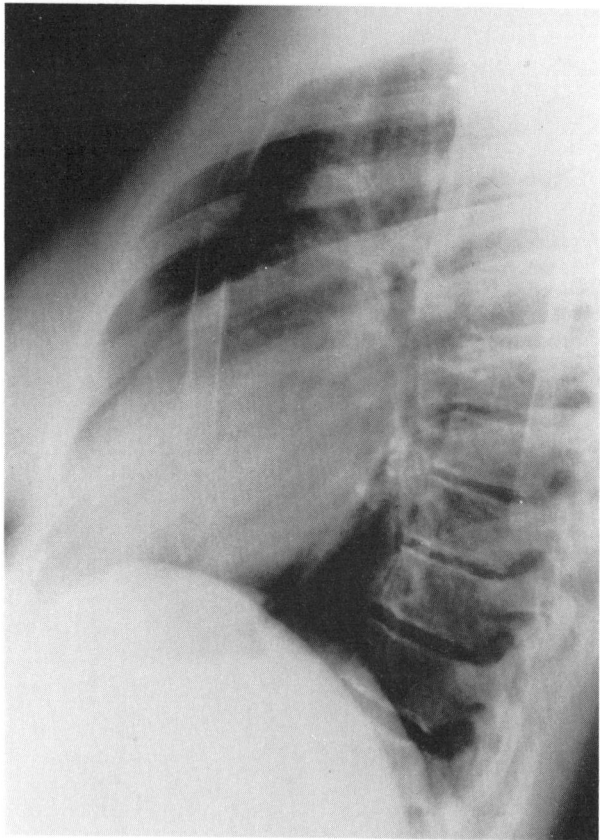

Fig. 72

Case 39

A 30-year-old Nigerian woman had the following chest X-ray. A close-up from the chest X-ray is also included (*Figs*. 73 and 74).

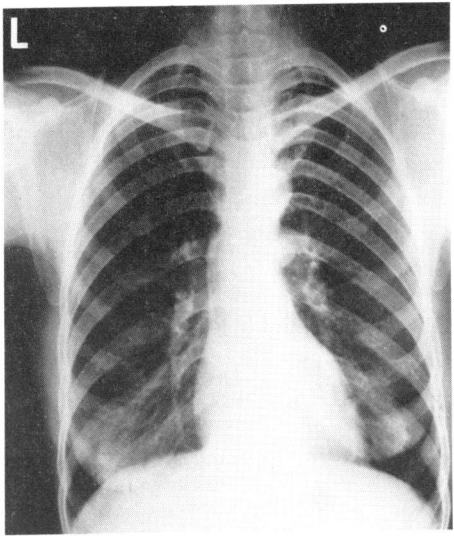

Fig. 74

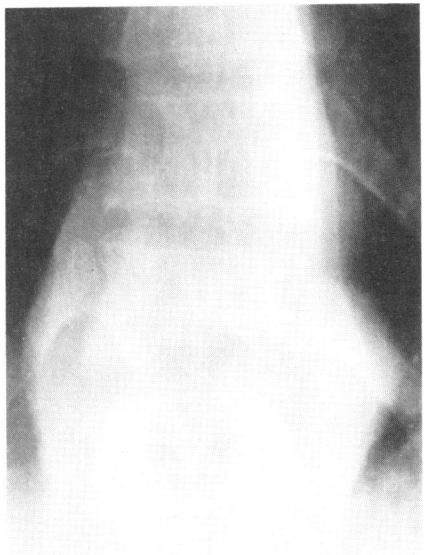

Fig. 73

Answer: Case 39

The heart and lungs appear normal. There is considerable widening of the paraspinal line bilaterally at the level of the diaphragm. Close examination reveals irregularity of the inferior margin of T12 and superior margin of Ll vertebral bodies and loss of height of the disc space. The appearances are thus those of a fusiform paraspinal mass with destruction of vertebral bodies and disc space narrowing. The causes of paravertebral opacities are listed in Table 39.1.

Table 39.1. Paraspinal masses

Neurogenic origin	— neurofibroma, neuroma
	— neuroblastoma
	— myelocoele and meningomyelocoele
Paravertebral abscess	— tuberculosis
	— pyogenic
	— brucellosis
Oesophageal	— hiatus hernia
	— achalasia
	— carcinoma
Metastases	— particularly from carcinoma of breast, bronchus, thyroid, kidney
	— myeloma and lymphoma
Aneurysm of descending aorta	
Pleural and pulmonary lesions adjacent to the vertebrae	— loculated pleural effusion
	— sequestrated lung segment
	— bronchogenic carcinoma
Primary bone tumour	— osteogenic sarcoma
	— aneurysmal bone cyst
	— chondrosarcoma
	— plasmacytoma
Extramedullary haemopoiesis	— thalassaemia
	— sickle cell
Sarcoidesis	
Oesophageal varices	— portal hypertension

Many of these conditions can be associated with bony abnormalities but the pattern of destruction either side of a narrowed disc space and fusiform swelling of soft tissues only occurs with infection.

Further questioning revealed a history of night sweats and weight loss and the final diagnosis of tuberculosis was made by needle biopsy.

Note on *Fig.* 73 the position of the side marker. The patient, in addition to the spinal tuberculosis, also has dextrocardia.

If you did not spot this remember the question 'what else?' Whenever you have spotted one abnormality on a film look also for others since there may be multiple-related or unrelated abnormalities—particularly on an examination film!

Case 40

A woman of 35 with cyanosis had the following chest X-ray (*Fig.* 75).

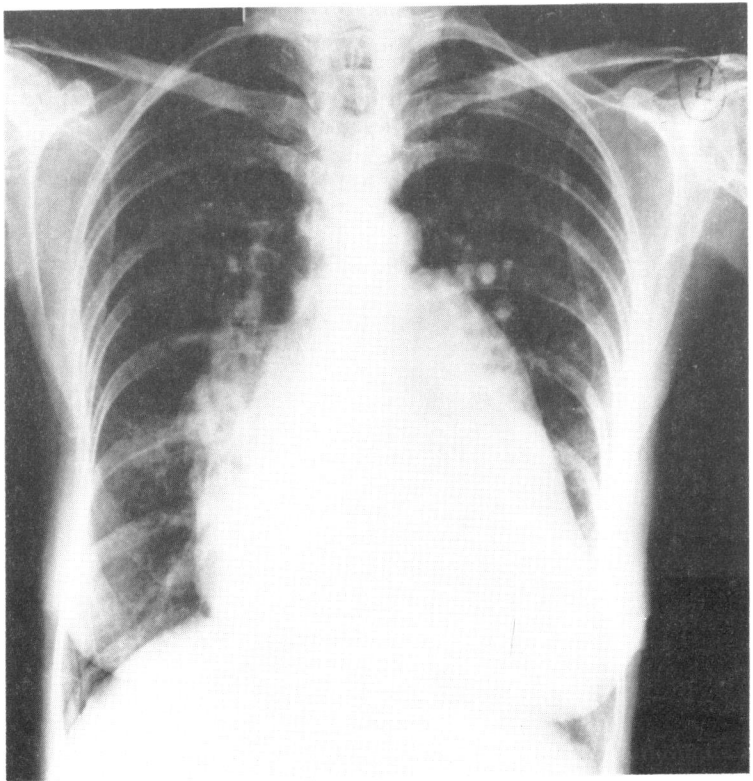

Fig. 75

Answer: Case 40

The heart is enlarged with marked enlargement of the main pulmonary artery. There is enlargement of proximal pulmonary arteries but the distal vessels are oligaemic and the lung fields are more radiolucent than normal.

The appearances are due to pulmonary arterial hypertension. This may be due to increase resistance to flow or to increased flow.

In this case the cause was an atrial septal defect. The peripheral oligaemia is due to pulmonary hypertension reversing the shunt. The subsequent right-to-left shunt leads to cyanosis. This is known as the Eisenmenger situation. At this stage it is not possible to close the ASD efficaciously and the only potentially curable treatment is heart–lung transplantation.

For more examples of cardiovascular disease see *Clinical Film Viewing in Cardiovascular Disease* by George Hartnell in the same series (Clinical Press, 1990).

Case 41

A woman, aged 84, had the following chest X-ray (*Fig.* 76).

What abnormality can be seen?

Which investigations may prove of value?

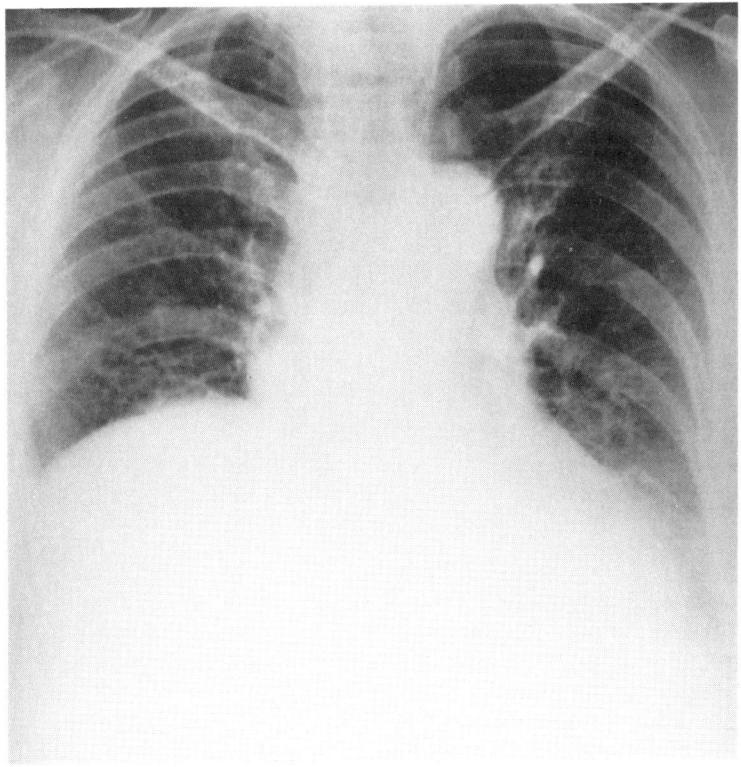

Fig. 76

Answer: Case 41

The right hemidiaphragm is raised. The heart is slightly enlarged. No definite lung lesion is seen. The hemidiaphragm may be raised because it is pulled up, pushed up, paralysed or simulated. The latter could be due to subpulmonary effusion or a mass abutting the diaphragm. Possible investigations include a right lateral film, lateral decubitus films, ultrasound and CT.

The lateral film (*Fig.* 77) shows the elevation of, the right hemidiaphragm to be partial, affecting the anterior part only. The ultrasound (*Fig.* 78) shows the liver immediately below the diaphragm. The anteromedial portion of the right cupola was thin compared with the more posterolateral part. There was no evidence of an effusion or mass.

The appearances are consistent with partial eventration of the diaphragm. The affected area is a thin fibrous sheet almost devoid of muscle fibres. Eventration is said to be asymptomatic without clinical significance but it must be distinguished from the other causes of elevation of the diaphragm. Complete eventration is said to be more common on the left side but partial eventration more commonly affects the right cupola.

Case 41

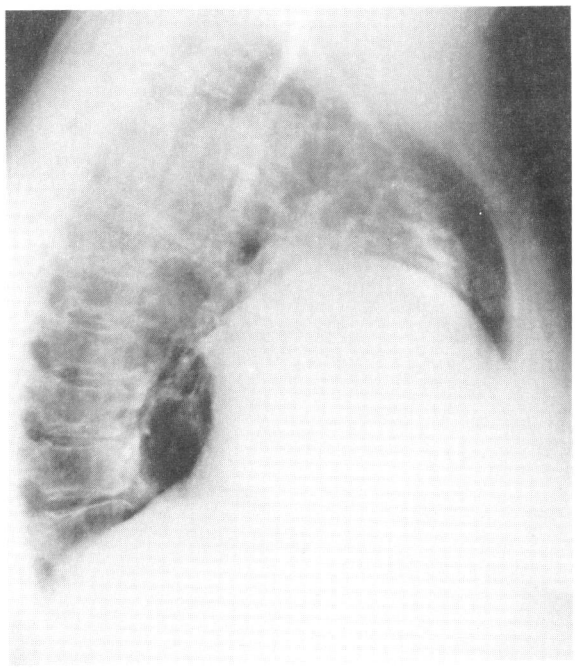

Fig. 77

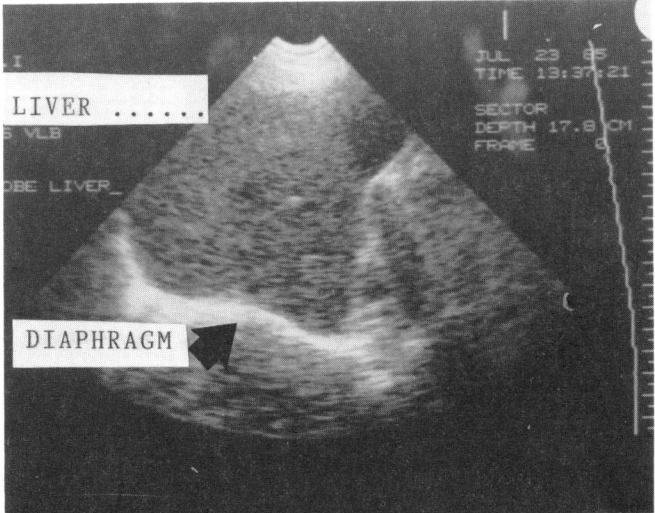

Fig. 78

Case 42

Woman, aged 58 (*Fig.* 79).

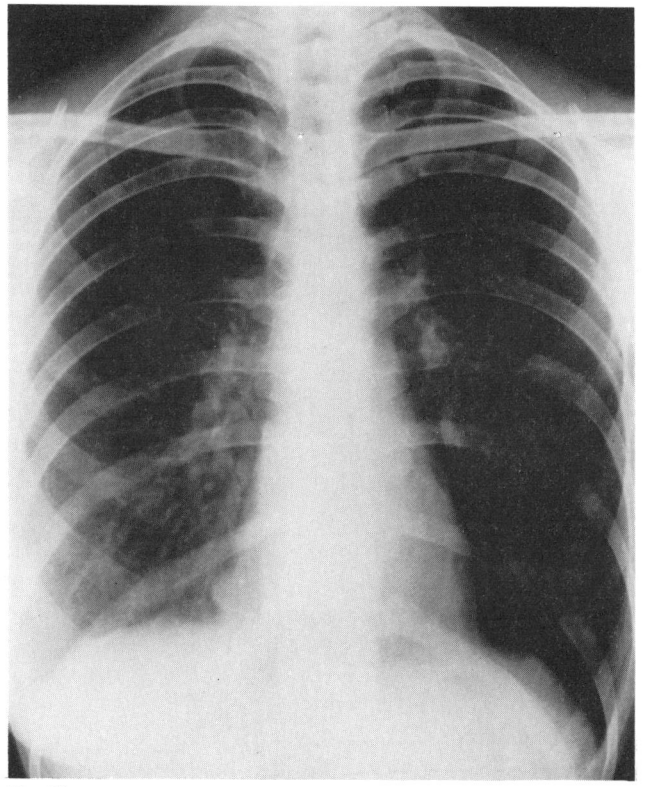

Fig. 79

Answer: Case 42

There is radiolucency of the left lung compared with the right. The right breast shadow is visible but the left is not and there has almost certainly been a mastectomy. The loss of soft tissue accounts for the difference in radiolucency.

A small rounded opacity is seen abutting the heart border in the right costophrenic angle. Further opacities are seen overlying the posterior aspect of the right 6th rib and in the left lung field.

In the presence of a mastectomy, secondary metastatic deposits from carcinoma of the breast are highly likely.

A flowchart for the investigation of unilateral translucency is reproduced as *Fig. 80*.

Conclusion

1. Left mastectomy.
2. Metastic deposits.

Table 42.1. Unilateral translucency of the chest

True decrease in density

1. Emphysema
   a. Compensatory emphysema
   b. Obstructive emphysema
   c. Bullous emphysema
   d. McLeod's (Swyer–James) syndrome
2. Pneumothorax
3. Cyst
4. Pulmonary emboli
5. Post-radiotherapy

Simulated

1. Rotation, scoliosis
2. Loss of soft tissue (mastectomy, Poland's syndrome)
3. Denser on the other side

From Goddard P. (1987) *Diagnostic Imaging of the Chest.* London, Churchill Livingstone.

Clinical Film Viewing

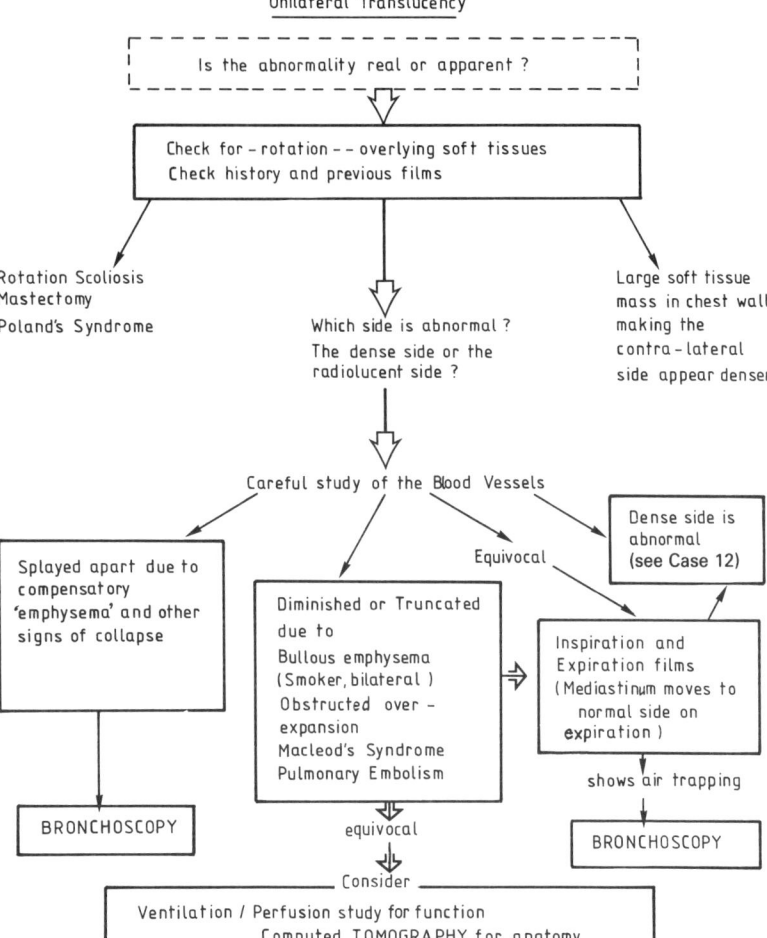

Fig. 80

Case 43

John presented in casualty looking very blue. His chest X-rays on inspiration and expiration are shown (*Figs.* 81, 82).

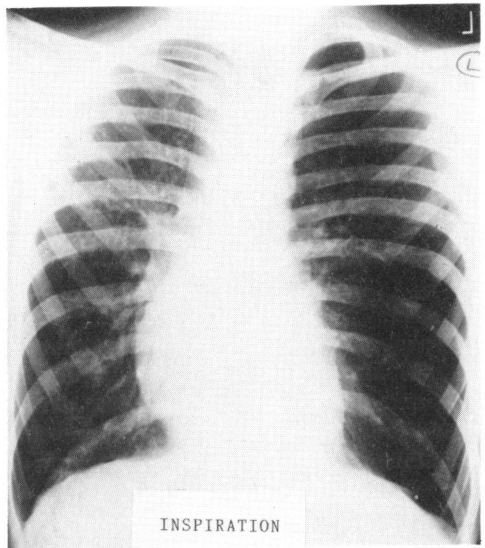

Fig. 81

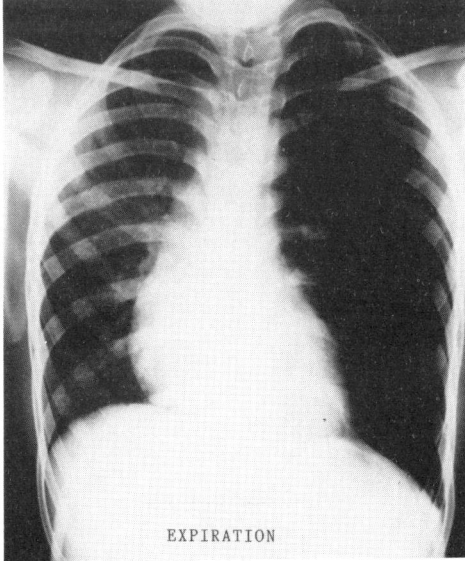

Fig. 82

Answer: Case 43

There is increased radiolucency of the left lung field and marked shift of the mediastinum to the right, particularly on the expiratory film.

Unilateral radiolucency can be due to a large number of causes including increased density of the opposite side.

The shift of the mediastinum away from the radiolucent side on expiration confirms that the abnormality is in the left lung. The appearances are consistent with obstructive 'emphysema' (overexpansion). Obstruction of the bronchi can be due to lesions in the lumen, in the wall, or outside but impinging upon the bronchus.

John had earlier been eating peanuts at a party. Bronchoscopy revealed a large peanut in the left main bronchus. This was successfully removed.

Removal of peanuts can be difficult since they are liable to break up into small pieces. If they do they can lead to lipid pneumonia and subsequent bronchiectasis.

Case 44

Gordon, 78 years old, presented with leg and chest pain. His investigations are shown (*Figs. 83–84*).

Case 44

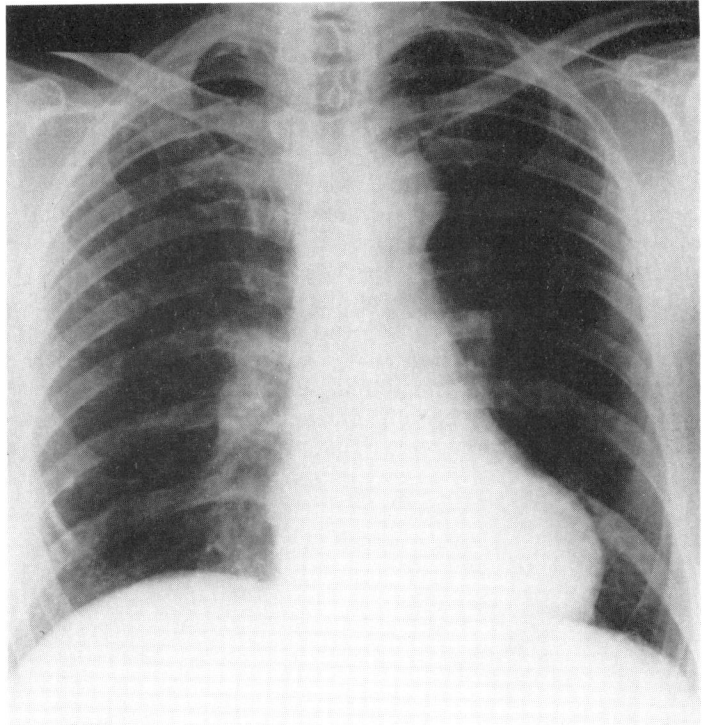

Fig. 83

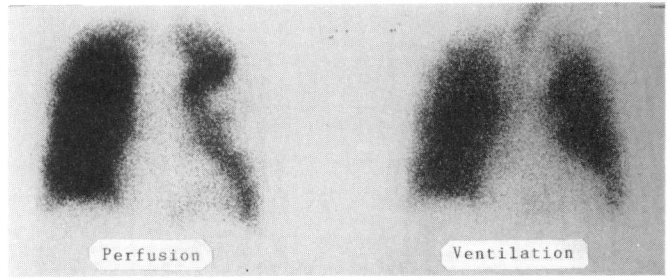

Fig. 84

Answer: Case 44

The heart size is within normal limits on the chest X-ray. There is relative translucency of the left mid zone compared with the right lung field. The right pulmonary artery is prominent.

The ventilation/perfusion study shows a large mismatched defect of perfusion in the left mid and lower zones. There is relatively increased perfusion in the right lung. The ventilation scan appears normal. In Bristol macroaggregates of albumin labelled with technetium-99m are injected intravenously for the perfusion study. Krypton-81m gas is used for ventilation studies, although in other centres xenon gas or an aerosol of technetium may be used.

The third study shown in *Figs*. 85 and 86 is a venogram of the right leg. Radiolucency is shown in the lumen of deep veins in the calf and thigh (arrowed). This represents thrombus.

Gordon had suffered from a pulmonary embolus following a deep vein thrombosis.

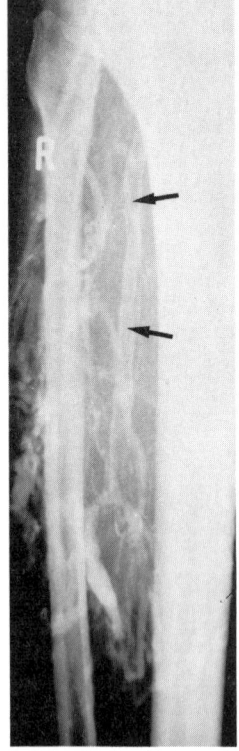
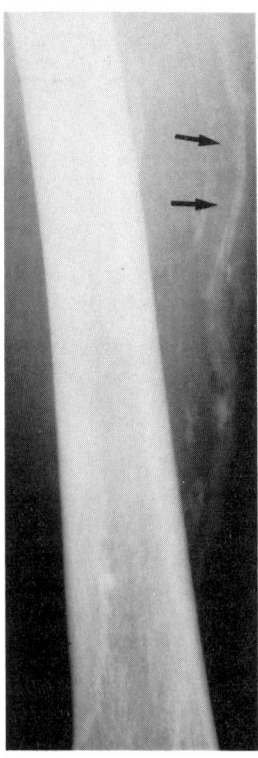

Fig. 85   *Fig*. 86

Case 45

A man, aged 45, with a history of light smoking, had the following chest X-ray (*Fig.* 87).

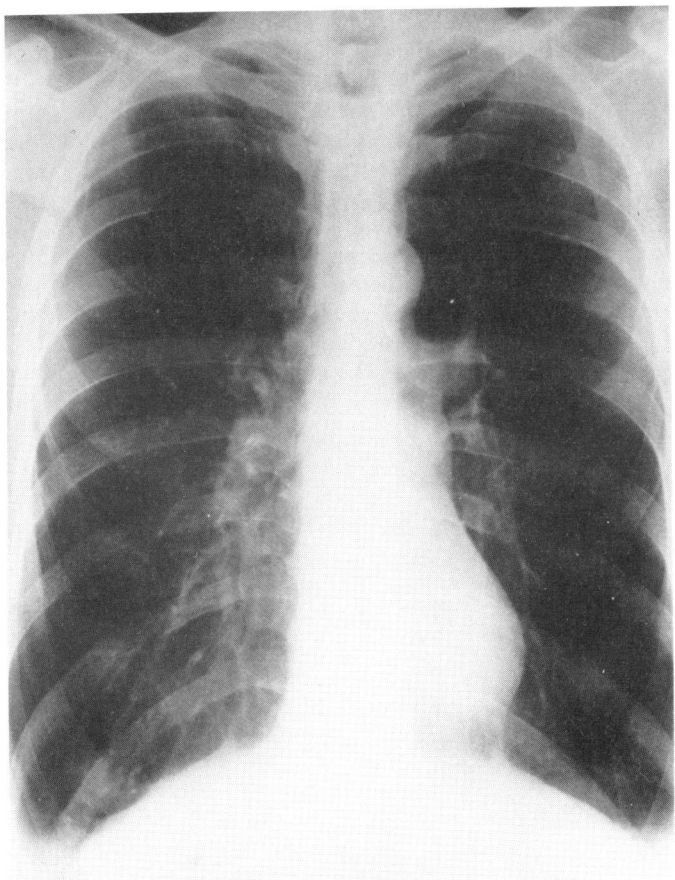

Fig. 87

Answer: Case 45

There is marked over-expansion of the lung fields associated with diminution in the vascularity. The appearances are those of pulmonary emphysema. At this age the possibility of alpha-1-antitrypsin deficiency must be considered. This condition is now known as alpha-1-antiprotease deficiency. The condition is characterized by predisposition to develop lung disease in the homozygote.

Fifty to sixty percent of homozygotes develop emphysema, often with marked cyanosis. Ten to twenty per cent develop liver disease. Emphysema develops by the fourth decade and is markedly worsened by smoking. Heterozygotes inherit the predisposition to develop emphysema especially if they smoke cigarettes.

The diagnosis of emphysema can be confirmed by CT scanning and by a low CO transfer factor. The emphysema in α-1-antiprotease deficiency tends to affect the lower zones initially. The diagnosis of α-1-antiprotease deficiency can be confirmed by demonstration of very low specific enzyme in the serum.

Reference

Eastham R. D. (1983) *A Laboratory Guide to Clinical Diagnosis.* Bristol, Wright, p. 208.

Case 46

A man, aged 55, was suffering from a chest infection that was not clearing on antibiotics (*Fig.* 88).

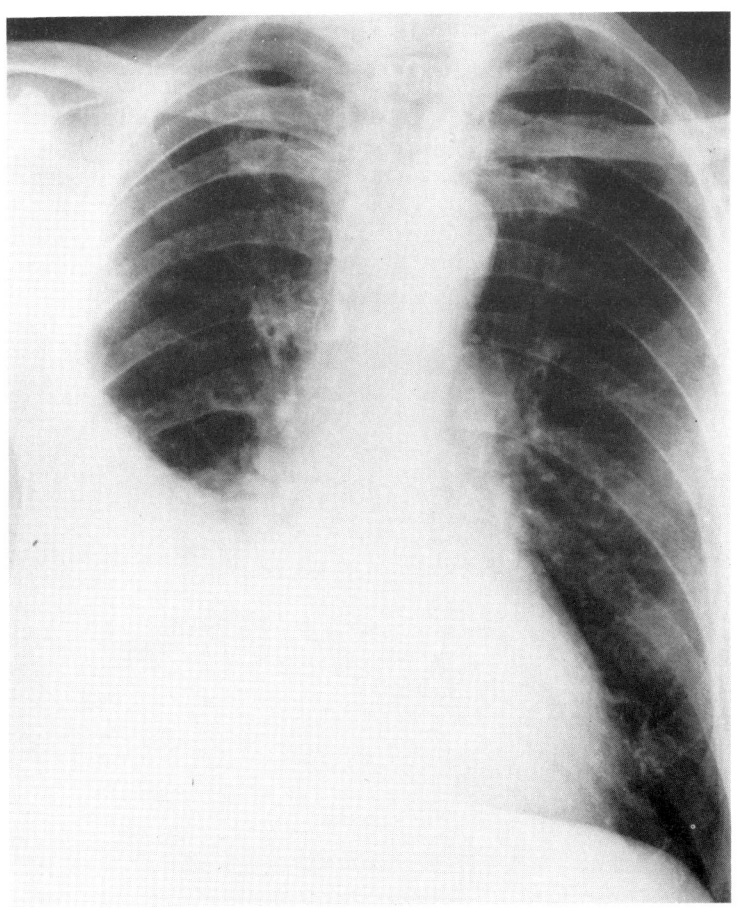

Fig. 88

Answer: Case 46

There is dense opacification in the right lower zone with obliteration of the right heart border and obscuring of the right hemidiaphragm. The opacity merges with a pleural shadow which could represent effusion or pleural thickening.

In view of the lack of response to antibiotics the possibility of empyema was considered. Ultrasound of the right lung field showed fluid-containing scattered echoes—ultrasound-guided aspiration yielded turbid fluid that grew *Streptococcus milleri* (*Fig.* 89).

The patient was referred to the chest surgeons who drained the empyema by means of a wide-bore tube.

A flowchart for the investigation of a pleurally based opacity is shown (*Fig.* 90). (*See also* Case 16 for investigation of persistent consolidation.)

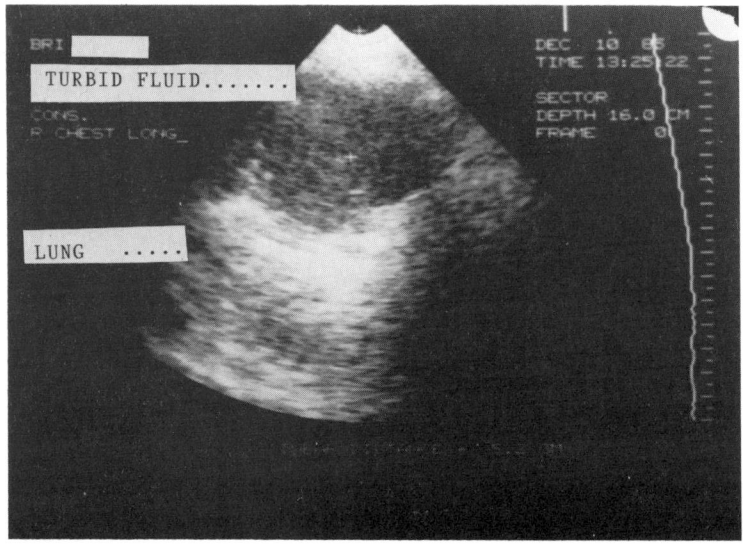

Fig. 89

Case 46

Pleurally Based Opacity

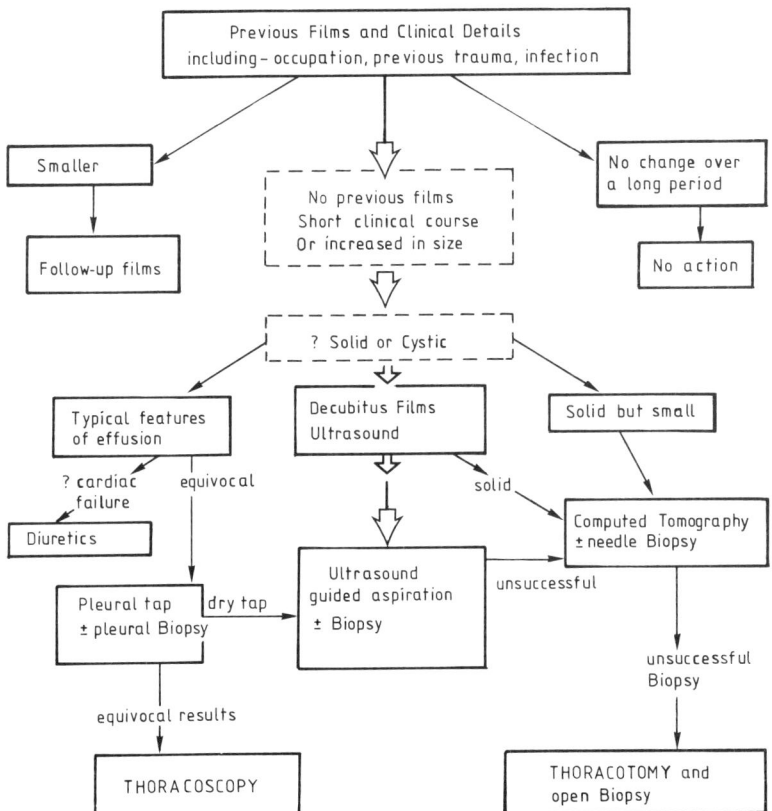

Fig. 90

Case 47

Malcolm, aged 60, was a Scottish plumber. He presented with a history of breathlessness. He had no other symptoms or signs. Two films from a series of chest X-rays are shown (*Figs*. 91 and 92).

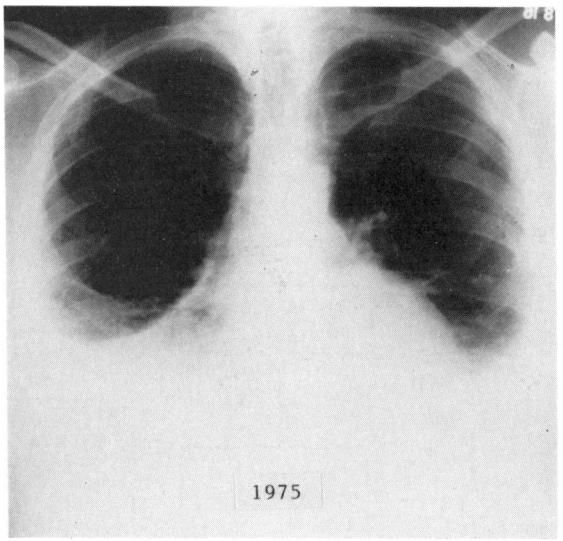

Fig. 91

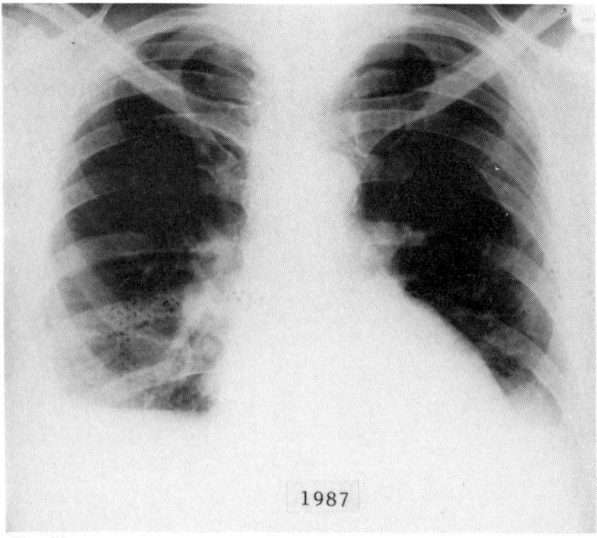

Fig. 92

Answer: Case 47

The first X-ray shows bilateral pleural effusions. Even in the absence of pyrexia, tuberculosis must be considered. Other possibilities initially considered included connective-tissue disorders (rheumatoid arthritis, SLE), infarction, pleural malignancy (primary or secondary) and pulmonary infection.

A pleural tap and pleural biopsy were performed. This revealed straw-coloured fluid containing very few cells and no organisms. Tuberculin test was only weakly positive and tests for rheumatoid factor and antinuclear factor were negative.

Further questioning of the patient revealed that he had a past occupational history of working as a lagger and had considerable exposure to asbestos.

Asbestos bodies were found in the patient's sputum. Benign pleural effusions are not uncommon due to asbestos exposure.

The second film showed bilateral pleural thickening.

Case 48

Valentina, aged 74, had stony dullness to percussion in the left lower zone and had the following chest X-ray (*Fig.* 93).

Report and suggest further investigation.

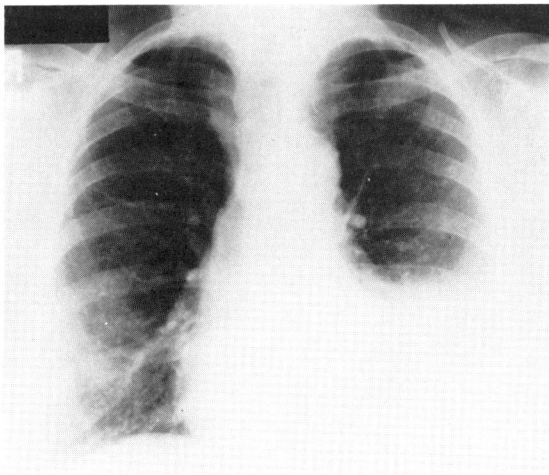

Fig. 93

Answer: Case 48

There is opacification in the left lower zone. The left heart border is obscured and the opacification merges with the left chest wall. The apppearances are consistent with a pleural effusion.

This could radiologically be confirmed by decubitus films, ultrasound or computed tomography but clinically the next investigation should be aspiration for cytology and culture. Pleural biopsy may also be performed at this time.

Aspiration revealed bloodstained fluid but nothing else of note.

The possibility of pulmonary embolism and infarction was considered and a ventilation/perfusion study undertaken (*Figs.* 94 and 95).

Ventilation/Perfusion Study (posterior (*Fig.* 94), posterior oblique (*Fig.* 95)):–

There is a large matched defect in the left lower zone and *better* perfusion than ventilation. This is consistent with the presence of a large effusion.* There is generalized matched reduction in the left mid and upper zones. The appearances do not support the diagnosis of pulmonary embolism but the result must be considered equivocal.

Subsequent clinical history was consistent with pulmonary infection.

Reference
* Goddard, P., Henson, J. and Davies, E. R. (1986) Pleural effusion causing unmatched ventilation defects in ventilation and perfusion scanning, *Clinical Radiology* **37**, 285–286.

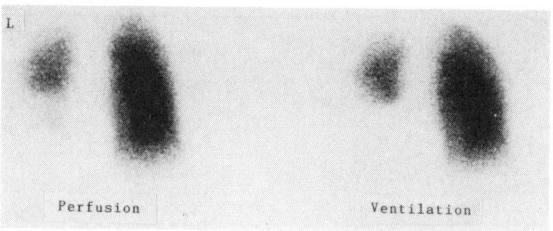

Fig. 94

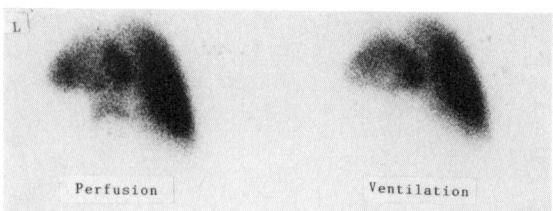

Fig. 95

Case 49

Mr Johnson, aged 55, had a chest X-ray because he had felt generally unwell for some time.

The chest X-ray is shown with close-up views of the left mid-zone and left hemidiaphragm (*Figs.* 96, 97 and 98).

What abnormalities are shown?

How should this be further investigated?

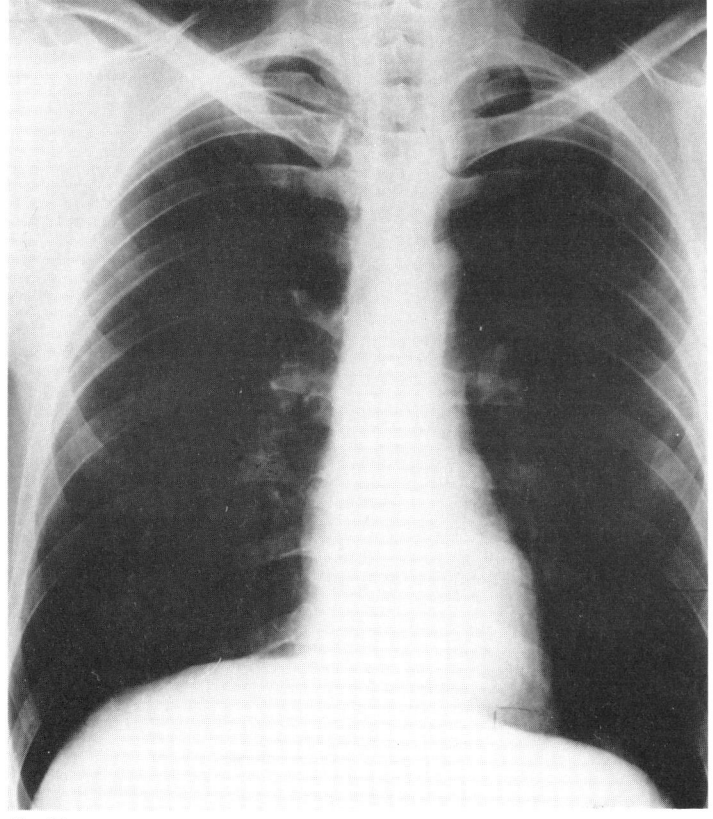

Fig. 96

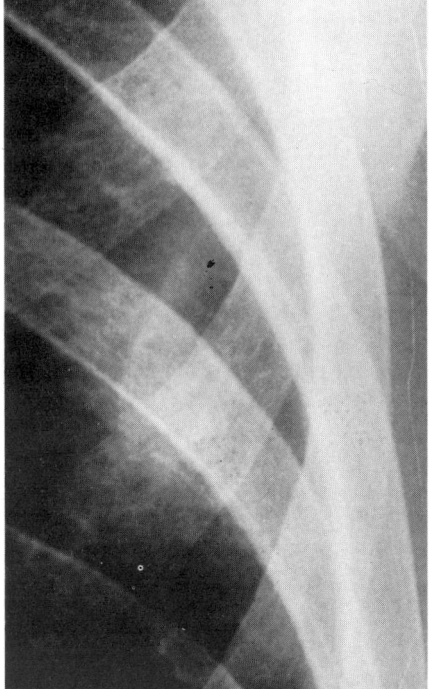

Fig. 97

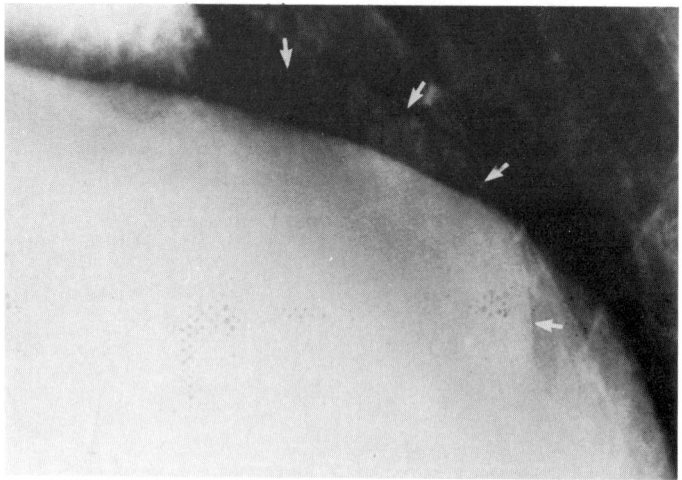

Fig. 98

Answer: Case 49

There is an ill-defined linear opacity peripherally in the left mid-zone. There is a further rounded opacity in the left lower zone—this has a 'setting sun' appearance and is of low density compared with the left hemi-diaphragm, which it is seen to overlap (the opacity has been arrowed on *Fig.* 98). No other abnormality is seen.

The mid-zone opacity is very peripheral and may well be pleural. Pulmonary abnormality cannot, however, be excluded. The lower zone mass is very smooth in outline and whilst it could be carcinoma it is more likely to represent a lipoma, fibroma, neurofibroma or cyst. In view of its low density a lipoma is most likely.

Computed tomography is the best investigation for the mid-zone opacity and for the lower zone mass.

Representative scans are shown in *Figs.* 99–101.

The CT scans revealed pleural plaques in the left mid-zones (arrowed on *Figs.* 99 and 100) and also in the right hemithorax. These are undoubtedly due to the asbestos exposure. the lower zone mass (*Fig.* 101) is shown to consist entirely of fat and is therefore a subpleural lipoma (density in Hounsfield units measured an average of -90).

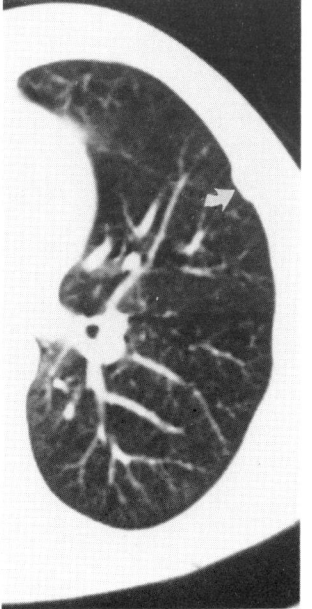

Fig. 99

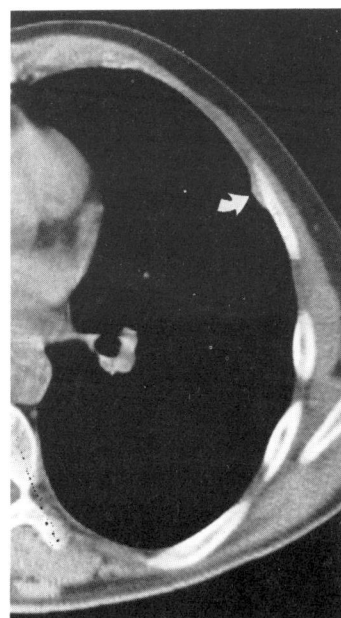

Fig. 100

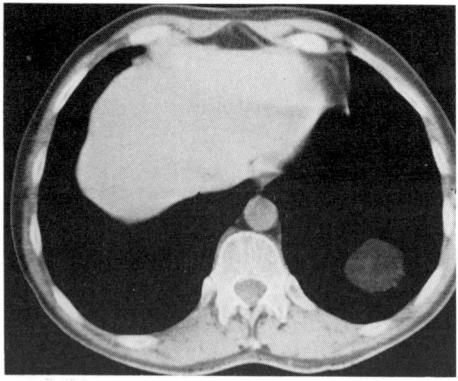

Fig. 101

Case 50

Charlotte, aged 12, presented with a painless lump on the lower part of the right side of the chest. Physical examination revealed a temperature of 38°C. (*Fig.* 102.)

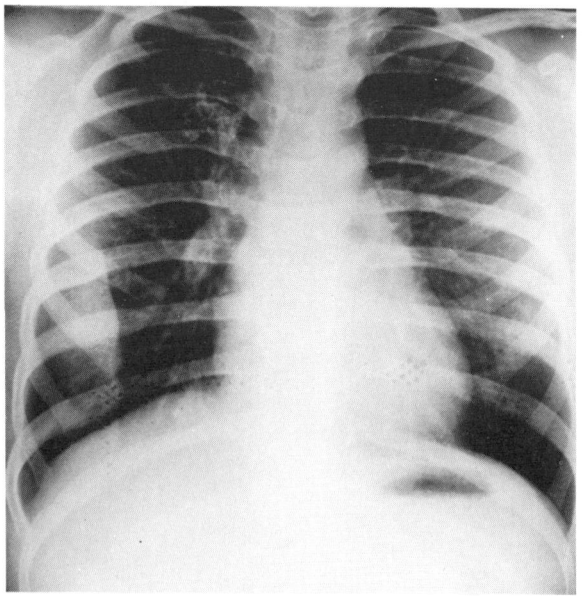

Fig. 102

Answer: Case 50

There is an opacity projected over the right hemithorax. The medial border is very distinct but the outer border and the superior border are not clearly seen.

There is a calcified opacity just superior to the right hilum. In addition there is erosion of the superior surface of the right 10th rib on the posterior aspect.

An 'incomplete border' is often present in lesions outside the lungs but projected over the lung field. It is frequently seen with pleural and chest wall masses. In this case fluoroscopy confirmed that the majority of the mass was subcutaneous but a pleural component was also demonstrated.

A mass in this site could represent:

1. An abscess — either tuberculosis, pyogenic or possibly actinomycosis.
2. Tumour — e.g. rhabdomyosarcoma (but rare in this site).
3. Haematoma.

The only diagnosis discussed above which could explain the calcified pulmonary lesion is tuberculosis.

The Mantoux reaction was strongly positive to 1:1000.

A large abscess involving the right latissimus dorsi was drained and a portion of the right 12th rib resected. Histology confirmed tuberculosis granulation tissue.

Case 51

Baby Matthew was breathless from birth but became acutely more breathless two hours before this chest X-ray was taken (*Fig.* 103).

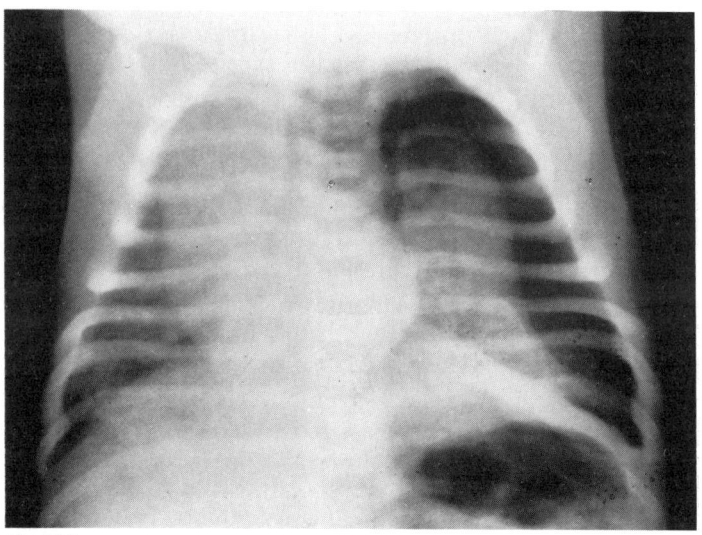

Fig. 103

Answer: Case 51

There is a radiolucent band in the left hemithorax and the cardiothymic shadow is shifted to the right. The left lung outline is clearly demarcated and no lung markings are seen within the radiolucency.

Both lungs are rather dense with the left lung denser than the right.

The appearances are due to a left-sided pneumothorax. The left lung has not completely collapsed but the heart is displaced to the right indicating a rise in intrapleural pressure.

Comment

In the neonate pneumothorax may result from obstruction due to aspirated blood or amniotic fluid or due to artificial ventilation.

The lungs often do not collapse completely and the air may be loculated anteriorly making visualization difficult. A horizontal beam lateral film or oblique films may help.

In older patients, pneumothorax may be more clearly shown by a film on expiration.

Case 52

Martin, a newborn premature baby, was cyanosed from birth. The chest X-ray 24 hours after birth is shown (*Fig.* 104).

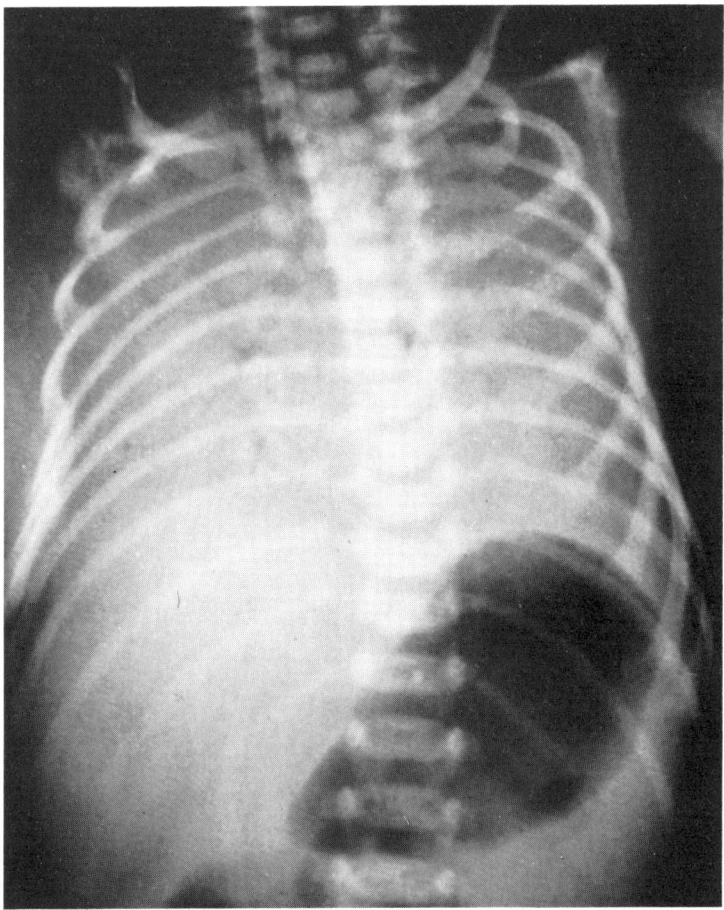

Fig. 104

Answer: Case 52

There is confluent shadowing in both lung fields. In the right lung field there is a branching pattern of linear radiolucencies. This is a sign known as an 'air bronchogram' and is seen when the alveoli are opacified due to a severe degree of hyaline membrane disease which is otherwise known as 'respiratory distress syndrome of the newborn'.

Table 52.1. Some causes of respiratory distress in the newborn

Respiratory distress syndrome
Pneumonia
Pulmonary haemorrhage
Brain damage—cerebral haemorrhage
Apnoea attacks
'Wet lung' (transient tachypnoea of the newborn)
Meconium aspiration
Pleural effusion
Pneumothorax
Congenital heart disease and cardiac failure
Oxygen toxicity
Bronchopulmonary dysplasia
Pulmonary agenesis or hypoplasia
Diaphragmatic hernia
Tracheo-oesophageal fistula

Comment

The radiological features of respiratory distress syndrome evolve over hours and days—first appearing within the first 12 hours. Serial films may therefore be valuable.

Case 53

An 11-year-old girl presented with recurrent cough, associated in the previous few days with vomiting, chest pain, dyspnoea and a small haemoptysis. Physical examination revealed pallor, tachycardia and tachypnoea with scattered râles over both lung fields (*Fig.* 105).

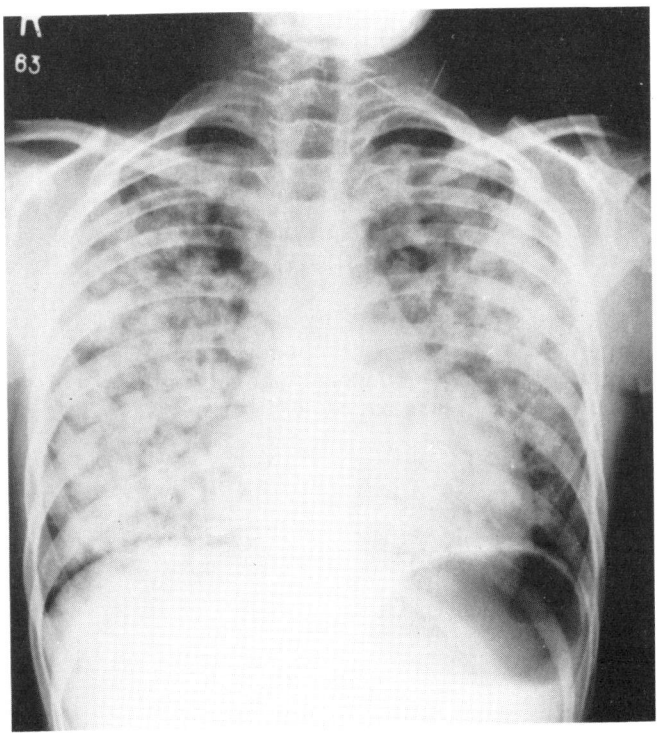

Fig. 105

Answer: Case 53

The chest X-ray shows widespread dense but ill-defined opacities which are confluent. There are irregular branching radiolucensies (air bronchograms). The heart is slightly enlarged.

The appearances are those of widespread alveolar opacification. In view of the heart size, pulmonary oedema must be considered and, with a history of haemoptysis, pulmonary haemorrhage. The latter is the more likely in view of the density of the opacification.

Urine contained casts and 35 red cells per high power field. There was severe anaemia and considerably raised urea. A massive haematuria was followed by a cardiac arrest from which she died.

Autopsy revealed extensive pulmonary haemorrhage both old and recent and evidence of progressive glomerulonephritis with crescent formation—this had probably been present for several months.

This case has the major features of Goodpasture's syndrome (widespread pulmonary haemorrhage, anaemia, progressive nephritis).

Goodpasture's syndrome was first described in 1919 and is due to an autoimmune response with antibodies against basement membranes in the pulmonary and glomerular capillary bed.

It is normally seen in young adult males and it is very rare under the age of 16.

Case 54

Luke, aged 12, had a short history of lassitude and cough. He was afebrile. (*Fig.* 106).

What are the possible causes in this age group?

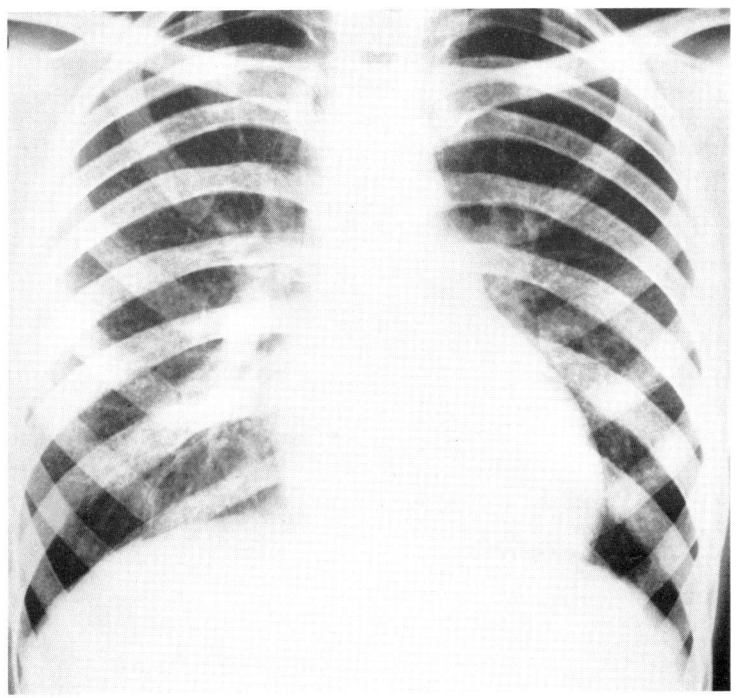

Fig. 106

Answer: Case 54

There are innumerable small nodules throughout both lung fields but predominantly in the mid-zones. The nodules are all of the same size (around 2 mm). No other abnormality is seen.

Conclusion

Widespread 'miliary' nodularity
In a child the causes of miliary nodularity have a different order of likelihood than in an adult, but the most important cause remains miliary TB, not because it is necessarily the most common but because it is eminently treatable but, untreated, may be readily fatal.

Table 54.1. Causes of miliary nodularity in a child and newborn

Child
Tuberculosis
Viral pneumonia
Allergic alveolitis
Cystic fibrosis
Histiocytosis-X
Gaucher's disease
Tuberose sclerosis
Sarcoidosis (from 12 years upwards)
Newborn
Respiratory distress syndrome (hyaline membrane disease)
'Wet lung' (transient tachypnoea)
Cardiac failure and pulmonary oedema
(e.g. due to total anomalous pulmonary venous drainage).
Acute bronchiolitis
Lymphangiectasia

(*See also* Case 22 for the causes of miliary nodularity in an adult.)

Further careful history taking revealed that Luke's father was a pigeon breeder and that Luke assisted him in his endeavours. Serology revealed high avian antibody titres confirming the diagnosis of allergic alveolitis or 'bird-fancier's lung'.

Case 55

A girl, aged 6, presented with lassitude and weight loss for six weeks and a dry cough for two weeks (*Fig.* 107).

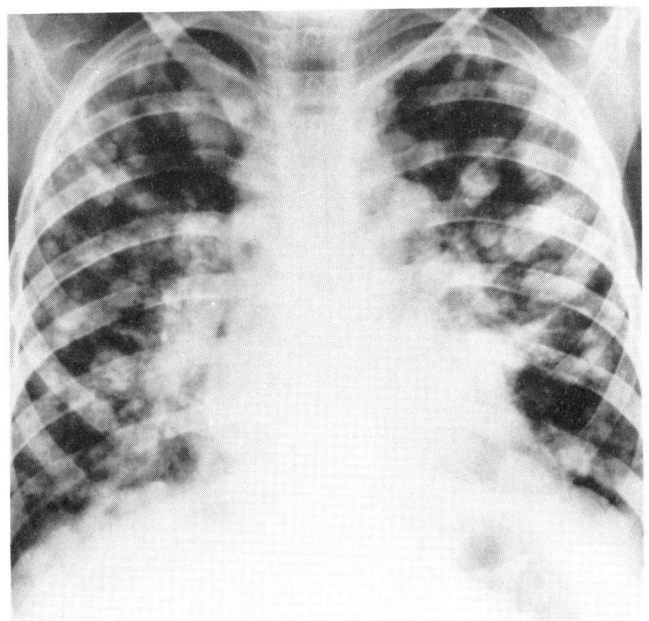

Fig. 107

Answer: Case 55

The chest X-ray shows multiple rounded opacities in both lung fields. The opacities vary in size. Possibilities include metastatic disease and multiple abscesses.

Physical examination revealed no fever but a hard irregular mass was palpable in the left loin.

The excretion-urogram (IVP) showed a mass in the left upper pole displacing and distorting the renal pelvis. The appearances were these of a nephroblastoma (Wilms' tumour). The two most common abdominal tumours in childhood are the nephroblastoma (Wilms' tumour) and the neuroblastoma. Neuroblastomas characteristically metastasize to bone whilst the Wilms' tumour commonly metastasizes to the lungs.

Case 56

Angela, aged 12, a known asthmatic had a six months history of lassitude and cough. Her chest X-ray is shown in *Fig.* 108.

As part of a study of chronic pulmonary problems in childhood, MRI was undertaken (*Figs.* 109 to 112).

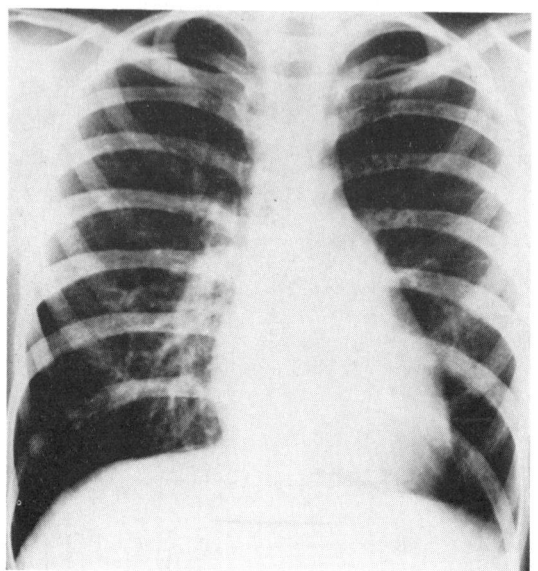

Fig. 108

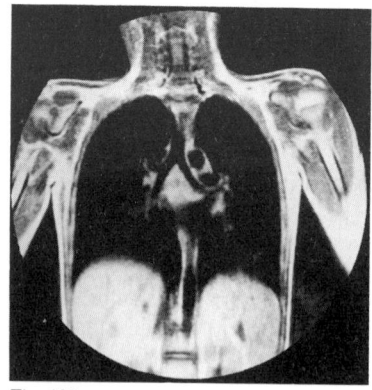

Fig. 109

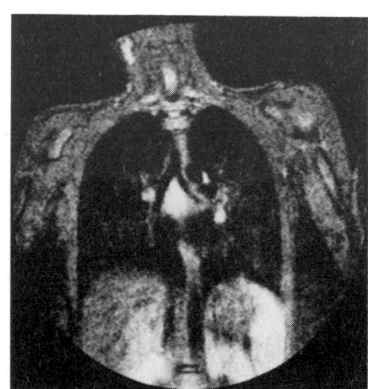

Fig. 110

Case 56

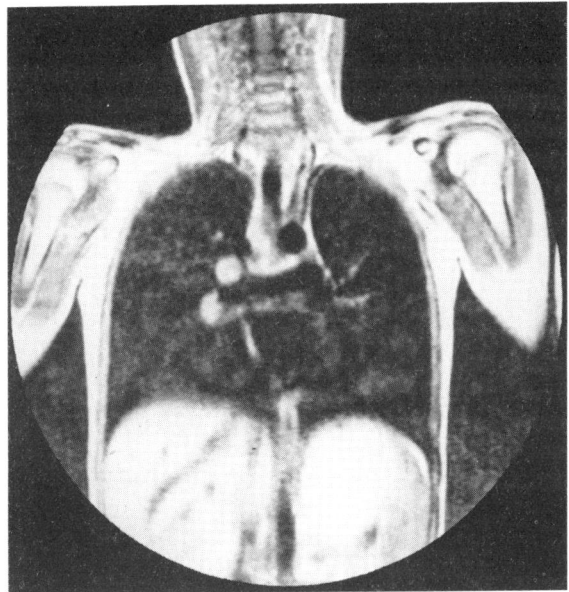

Fig. 111

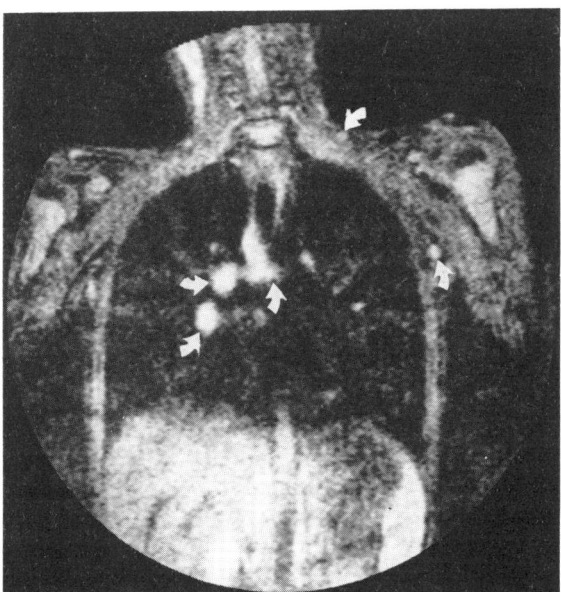

Fig. 112

Answer: Case 56

The heart size is within normal limits. There is a slight bulge in the region of the pulmonary artery but this was also considered to be normal. An increase in bronchovascular markings in the right lower zone could be due to asthma.

The MRI scans were obtained in the coronal plane using 'T1 weighted' and 'STIR' sequences. The 'T1-weighted' scans provide very good anatomical information. The 'STIR' sequence (Short Tau Inversion Recovery) is a technique that suppresses the signal from fat and highlights structures with a high water content. In this case the 'STIR' sequence highlights large nodes demonstrated on the T1 weighted scans. Typical lymph nodes are arrowed on *Fig.* 112. There are very large hilar nodes and subcarinal and paratracheal mediastinal nodes. There are smaller, but still enlarged, cervical and axillary nodes.

The spleen was also slightly enlarged. In an adolescent the possible causes of lymphadenopathy include lymphoma, leukaemia, infections such as infectious mononucleosis (glandular fever) and cat-scratch fever. Sarcoidosis can also occur in late childhood although it is uncommon at such a young age.

The reticuloses were considered unlikely due to the predominence of hilar node enlargement rather than upper mediastinal nodes. The most likely diagnosis was considered to be infectious mononucleosis and a positive Paul–Bunnell test proved this to be the case.

This example demonstrates the clarity of MRI in showing mediastinal structures. The subject of MRI is covered in two companion books in the *Clinical Film Viewing Series* (*An Introduction to Clinical MRI* and *CT and MRI Film Viewing*).

Case 57

Mabel, 73, presented with stridor. Her chest X-ray is shown (*Fig.* 113).

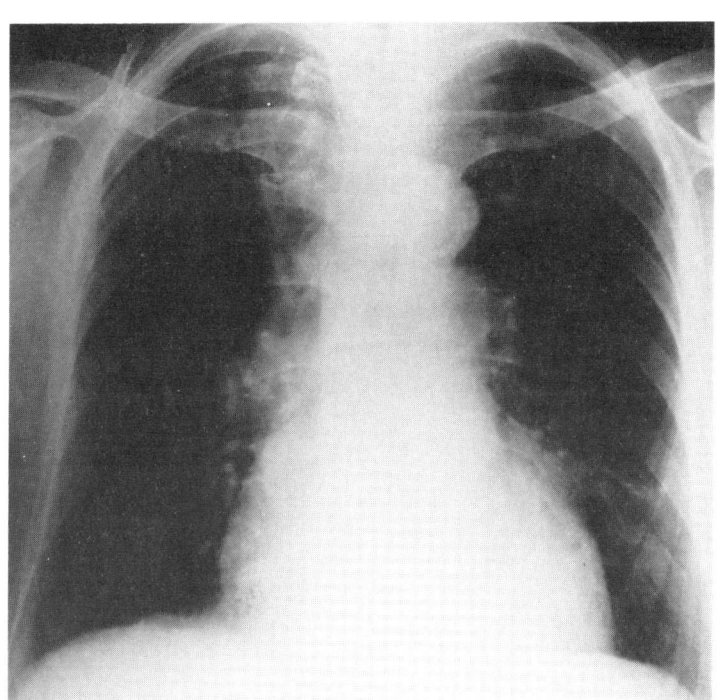

Fig. 113

Answer: Case 57

There is considerable widening of the superior mediastinum extending into the neck. There is calcification within the mass.

The heart is enlarged and there is calcification of the aorta.

CT (*Fig.* 114) confirms the presence of the superior mediastinal mass and shows focal calcification within the mass. There is considerable narrowing of the trachea. Further scans into the neck revealed that the mass was continuous with and indistinguishable from the thyroid gland.

The mass represented a large calcified nodular thyroid goitre. This was surgically excised and confirmed as benign in nature.

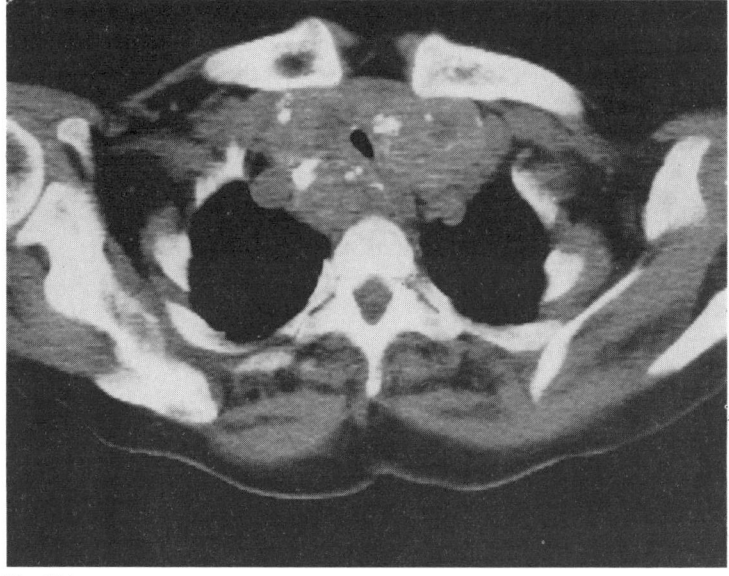

Fig. 114

Comment

This case and the following cases are revision material—the basic information has been covered in the preceding cases.

Case 58
Mr Burman, aged 57, had the following routine employment chest X-ray (*Fig.* 115).

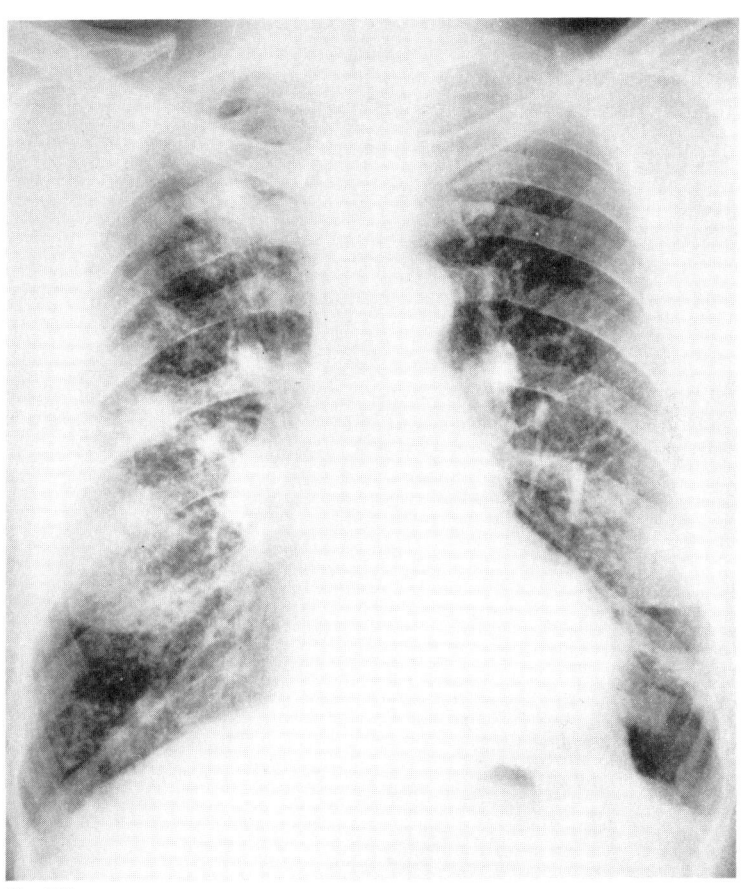

Fig. 115

Answer: Case 58

The chest X-ray showed the heart size to be normal. There are multiple nodules and lines throughout the lung fields. In addition there are more confluent areas of opacification in the right mid and upper zones. The opacities have irregular borders. There is no significant pleural component. The appearances are consistent with pneumoconiosis with progressive massive fibrosis.

Comment

Progressive massive fibrosis is typically described* as 'a poorly-defined shadow some 2–5 cm in diameter, commonly in the mid zone or just below the clavicle'. This is associated with the small circular shadows representing the basic nodule of the pneumoconiosis.

Reference

*Simon, G. (1978) *Principles of Chest X-ray Diagnosis,* 4th ed. London, Butterworths, pp. 125–127.

Case 59

A 65-year-old man suffering from pyrexia and productive cough had right basal crepitations (*Fig.* 116).

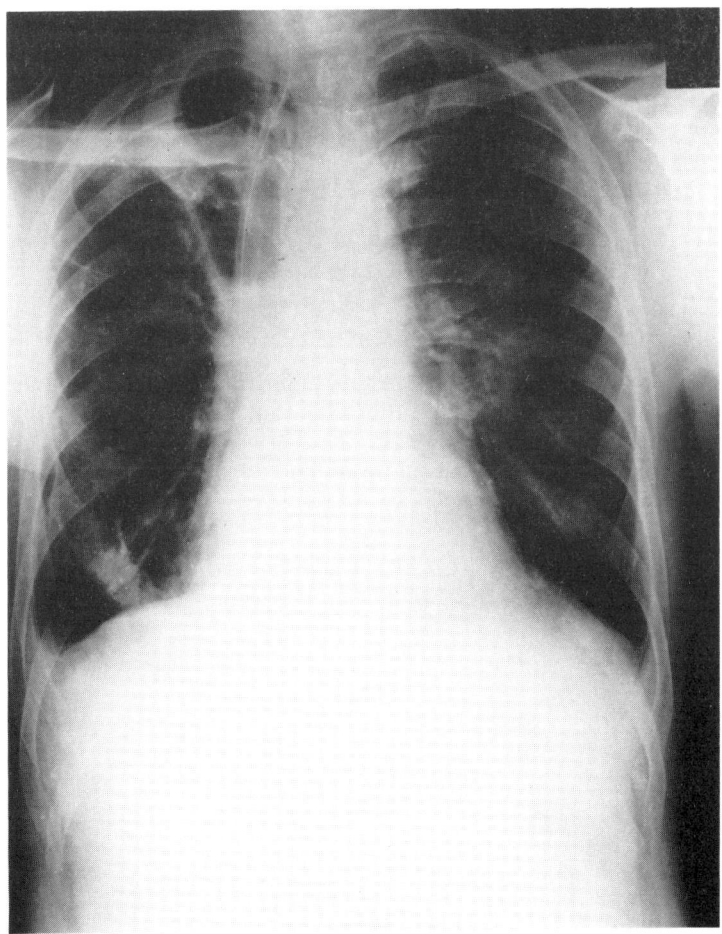

Fig. 116

Answer: Case 59

There is widening of the mediastinum and a fluid level within the mediastinum. A nasogastric tube can be seen with the tip in the mediastinum just below the fluid level. There is no stomach bubble under the left hemidiaphragm. There is patchy opacification adjacent to the left hilum and in the right lower zone and small bilateral pleural effusions.

The absence of a stomach bubble suggests:

    achalasia
    oesophageal carcinoma
    gastric pull-through operation

The fluid level in the mediastinum is in keeping with:

    oesopheageal dilatation
    gastric pull-through
    (rarely) mediastinal abscesses—gas-forming organisms

Inspection of the patient's history immediately revealed that he had undergone a gastric pull-through operation for oesophageal carcinoma.

The pulmonary opacification was due to inhalation and subsequent pneumonia.

Comment

The absent stomach bubble is an important sign (especially in exams)!

Case 60

Mr Langsdale, aged 50, had right-sided pleuritic chest pain and a palpable mass posteriorly on his chest wall. Chest X-ray showed hazy opacification in the right lower zone. CT is shown (*Figs.* 117–119).

Case 60

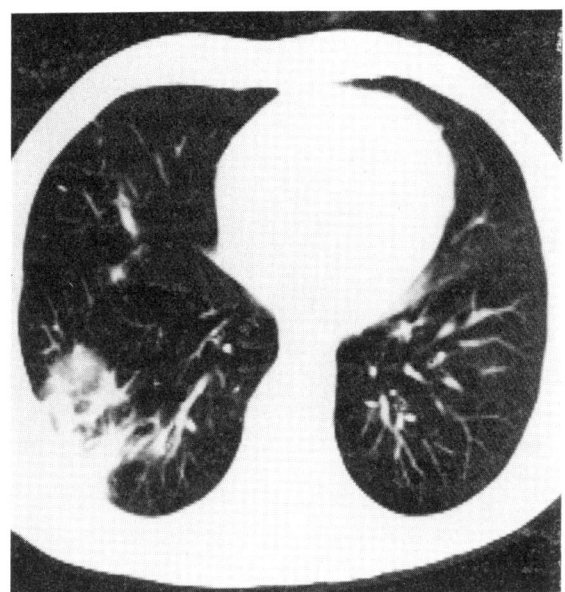

Fig. 117

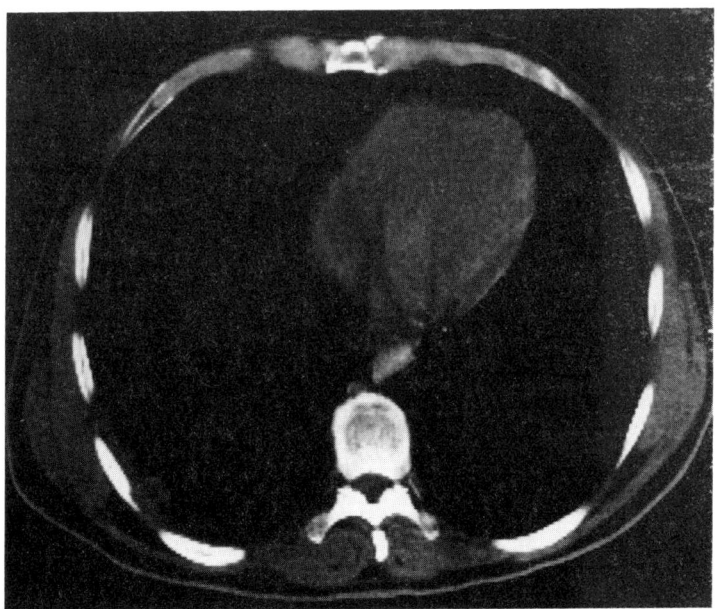

Fig. 118

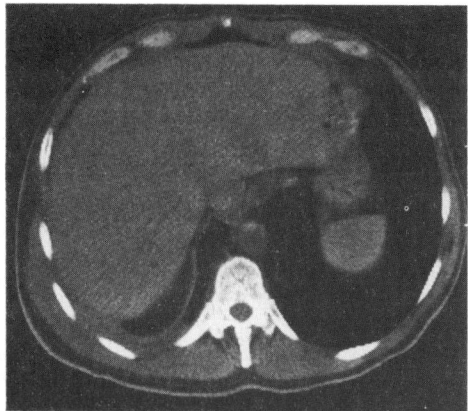

Fig. 119

Answer: Case 60

The CT shows ill-defined opacification peripherally in the right lung associated with pleural thickening. A soft-tissue mass is clearly shown on the more inferior scan.

The pulmonary opacification has the appearances of consolidation rather than a mass. Consolidation associated with pleural and chest wall lesions is unusual and actinomycosis should be considered.

Some malignant conditions, e.g. lymphoma, mesothelioma and carcinoma of the bronchus, can result in a similar combination of pulmonary, pleural and chest wall lesions.

The predominance of each component is, however, different. In lymphoma it is likely that there would be large mediastinal nodes. This is also true with carcinoma of the bronchus and in this condition the pulmonary abnormality is usually a mass or dense consolidation distal to a mass. Patients with mesothelioma have a predominantly pleural mass.

Periosteal new bone formation should be sought in those ribs adjacent to any large longstanding pleural or pulmonary shadow of unknown aetiology. A combination of consolidation and periostitis of overlying ribs will suggest a diagnosis of actinomycosis, although not visible on these scans and not on careful examination of the chest X-ray.

Pulmonary actinomycosis is a rare disease due to *Actinomyces israelii*. Pathologically it causes typical 'honeycomb' abscesses in the affected lung and involves adjacent chest structures. It is surrounded by a dense fibrous reaction with the fungus in the form of 'sulphur granules' in the pus.

(*See also* Case 50.)

Case 61

Napoleon B., aged 82, had the following chest X-ray and CT scan (*Figs.* 120 and 121).

Report on the chest X-ray?

What does the CT show?

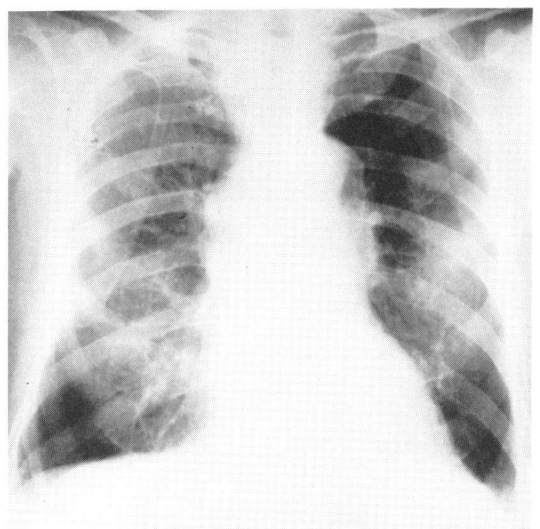

Fig. 120

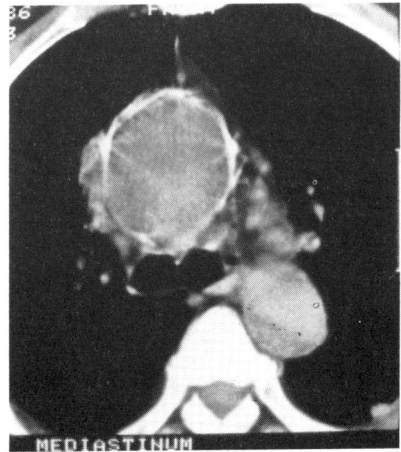

Fig. 121

Answer: Case 61

On chest X-ray the heart size is normal but there is marked mediastinal widening. No active lung lesion is seen.

CT of the mediastinum shows calcification of an aneurysm of the ascending aorta. The descending aorta appears normal.

The most common cause of a calcified aneurysm is an atheromatous aneurysm. In the absence of abnormality in the descending aorta, a syphilitic cause should be considered. Other important causes of aneurysms include traumatic rupture and dissection.

In this case there was a history of syphilis in 1922 and he was now suffering from syphilitic aortitis with a degree of aortic incompetence.

Cardiovascular problems are covered in great detail in *Clinical Film Viewing in the Cardiovascular System* by George Hartnell (Clinical Press).

Note that a pleural plaque is just visible on the CT scan posteriorly in the left hemithorax. A history of asbestos exposure was elicited and several plaques were seen on the set of scans.

Comment

Don't forget in the exam situation to think 'what else?' and look for extra lesions.

Case 62

Peter, aged 62, had a two-year history of worsening dyspnoea. He also had finger clubbing and pulmonary function studies showed a low transfer factor and vital capacity. (*Fig.* 122.)

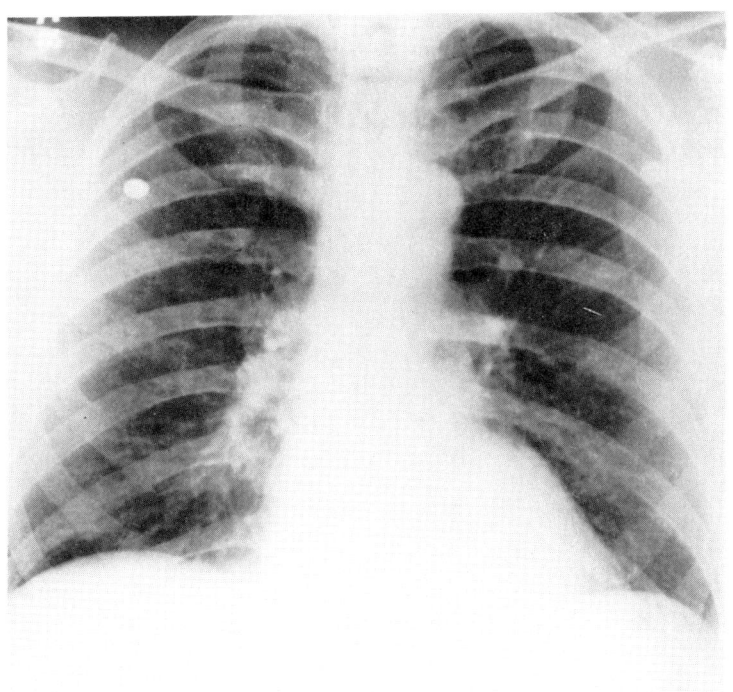

Fig. 122

Answer: Case 62

The heart size and shape are normal. There is a slight nodular opacification in both lower zones. Electrodes from ECG leads are noted. The nodular opacification is only slight and could be within normal limits but in view of the history further investigation, including CT is indicated.

A close-up of the right lower zone on the CT scan is shown in *Fig. 123*. This shows small peripheral ring structures and emphysematous bullae. The appearances are consistent with fibrosing alveolitis.

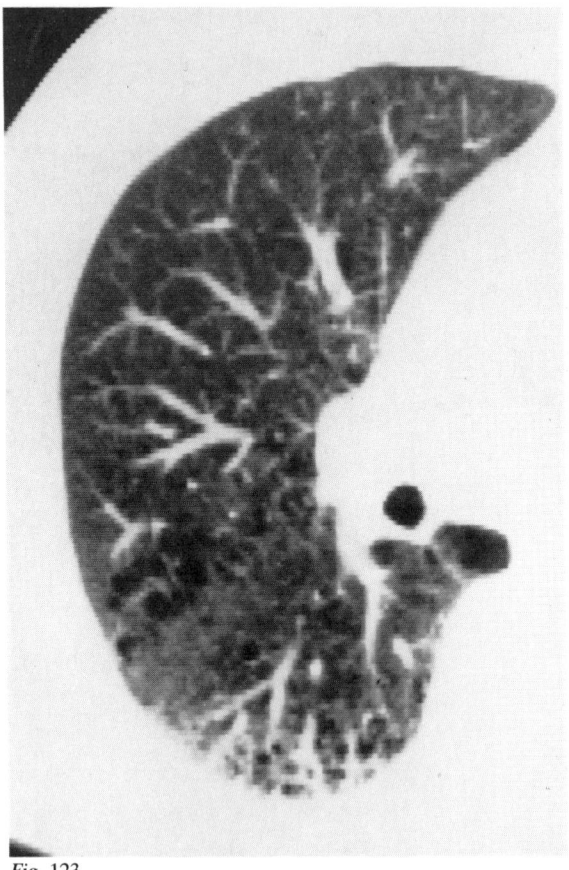

Fig. 123

Case 63

A 66-year-old man with symptoms of pneumonia had the following chest X-ray (*Fig.* 124).

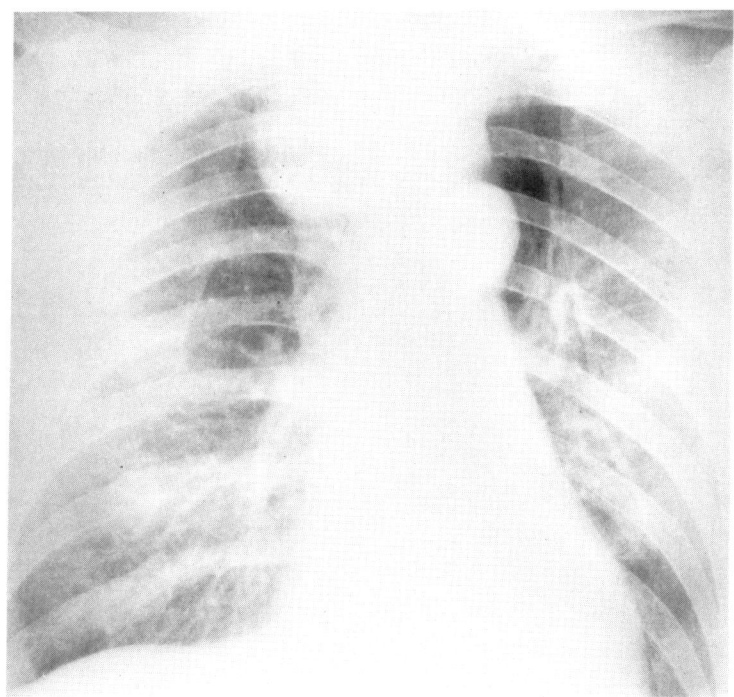

Fig. 124

Answer: Case 63

There is widening of the superior mediastinum with a smooth rounded outline. Further investigation may include computed tomography and biopsy. The lesion may either represent a mass from the mediastinum or a pulmonary mass abutting the mediastinum.

Following percutaneous needle biopsy a pneumothorax developed (*Fig.* 125). Pneumothorax occurs in between 10% and 30% of patients following percutaneous needle biopsy but only requires drainage in a small percentage.

In this case the pneumothorax has confirmed that the lesion lies in the apex of the right lung! Cytology showed poorly-differentiated malignant cells.

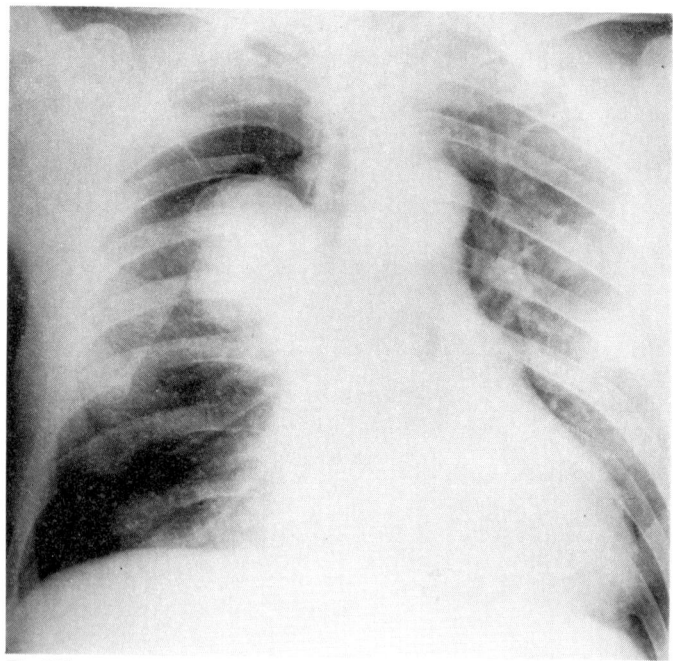

Fig. 125

Case 64

The chest X-ray of a man aged 33 (*Fig.* 126).

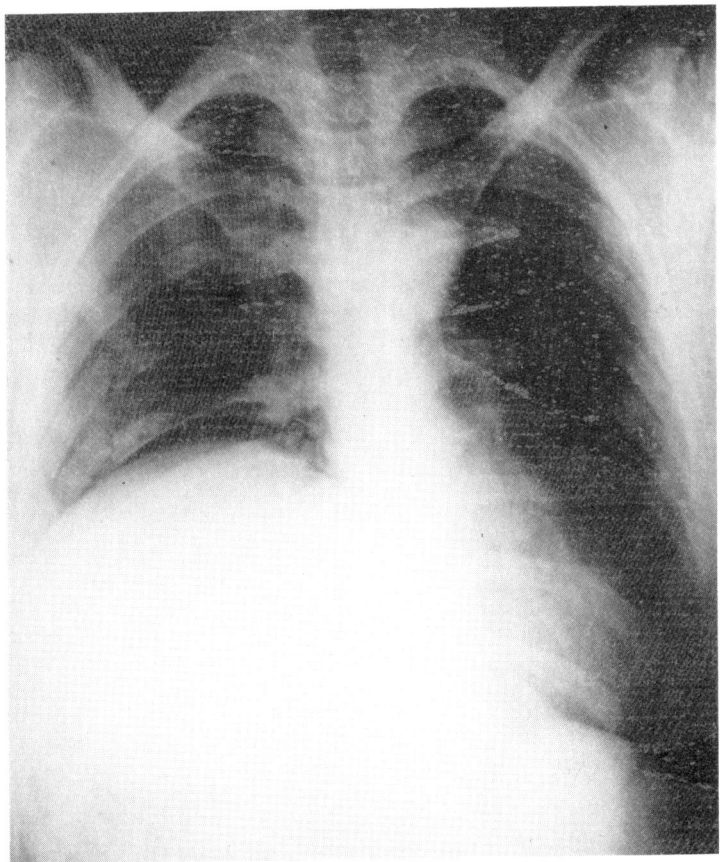

Fig. 126

Answer: Case 64

The right hemidiaphragm appears raised. In addition there are fractures of several of the right ribs, indicative of considerable trauma. The 'raised hemidiaphragm' may represent a subpulmonary pleural effusion due to haemorrhage (haemothorax) or diaphragmatic rupture with the liver in the right hemithorax. Differentiation may be made by decubitus films, ultrasound or CT.

Comment

In this case there was a traumatic rupture of the diaphragm. This is a life-threatening condition that may be catastrophically forgotten.

It can result in hernial bleeding or strangulation. If the hemidiaphragm is torn but herniation has not occurred, the only available radiological signs may be pneumoperitoneum or pneumothorax. There may be signs of associated trauma such as rupture of the liver or spleen. Barium studies may be helpful by showing herniation of gut and ultrasound, CT or MRI may show herniation of omentum, liver or other viscera.

Reference

Goddard, Paul R. (1987) *Diagnostic Imaging of the Chest.* London, Churchill-Livingstone.

Case 65

A woman, aged 60, had a 'routine' chest X-ray (*Figs*. 127 and 128).

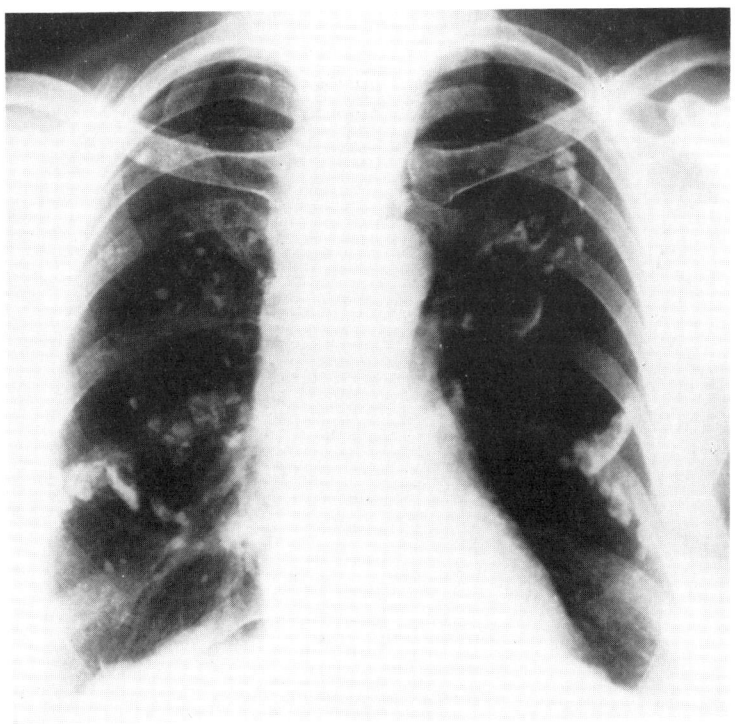

Fig. 127

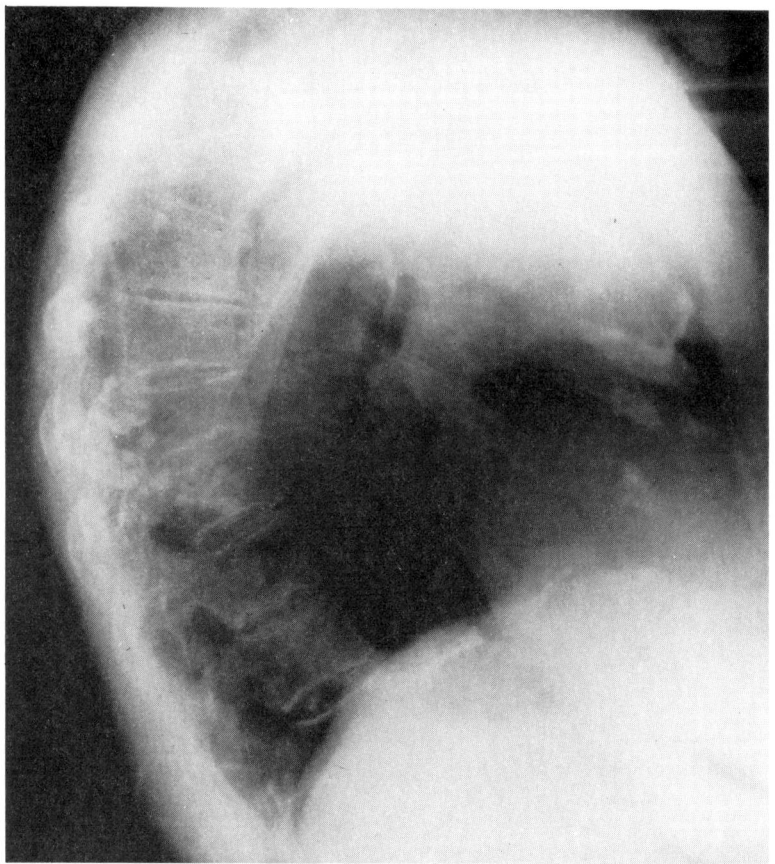

Fig. 128

Answer: Case 65

There is pleural calcification bilaterally. There is calcification over the diaphragm visible on the lateral film.

The appearances are due to calcification of pleural plaques following asbestos exposure. Degenerative spondylosis is noted in the thoracic spine.

Case 66

Graham, 25, had suffered from shortness of breath for a month or two. This had worsened recently. (*Fig.* 129)

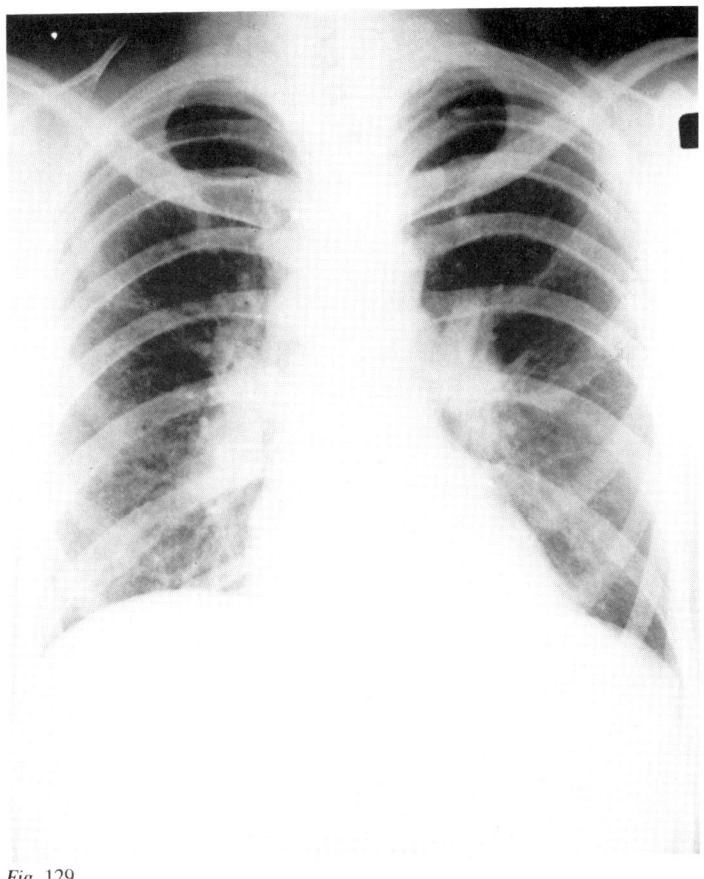

Fig. 129

Answer: Case 66

The chest X-ray shows enlargement of the hilar shadows bilaterally and slight nodularity in both lung fields. There is widening also of the mediastinum. The appearances are those or enlarged hilar and paratracheal lymph nodes. The appearances are classical of sarcoidosis.

Comments

Similar features can be seen in lymphoma although the distribution is more mediastinal than hilar in the reticuloses. Alternative diagnoses for bilateral hilar node enlargement are less likely but include berylliosis, cat-scratch fever and infectious mononucleosis.

In tuberculosis and carcinoma of the bronchus the lymph-node enlargement is usually unilateral. Enlarged pulmonary arteries can similarly enlarge the hila but the main pulmonary arteries would be prominent just below the aortic knuckle and the paratracheal region would not be involved.

The pulmonary opacification was also due to sarcoidosis.

Case 67

An asthmatic lady, 35 years of age. (*Fig.* 130.)

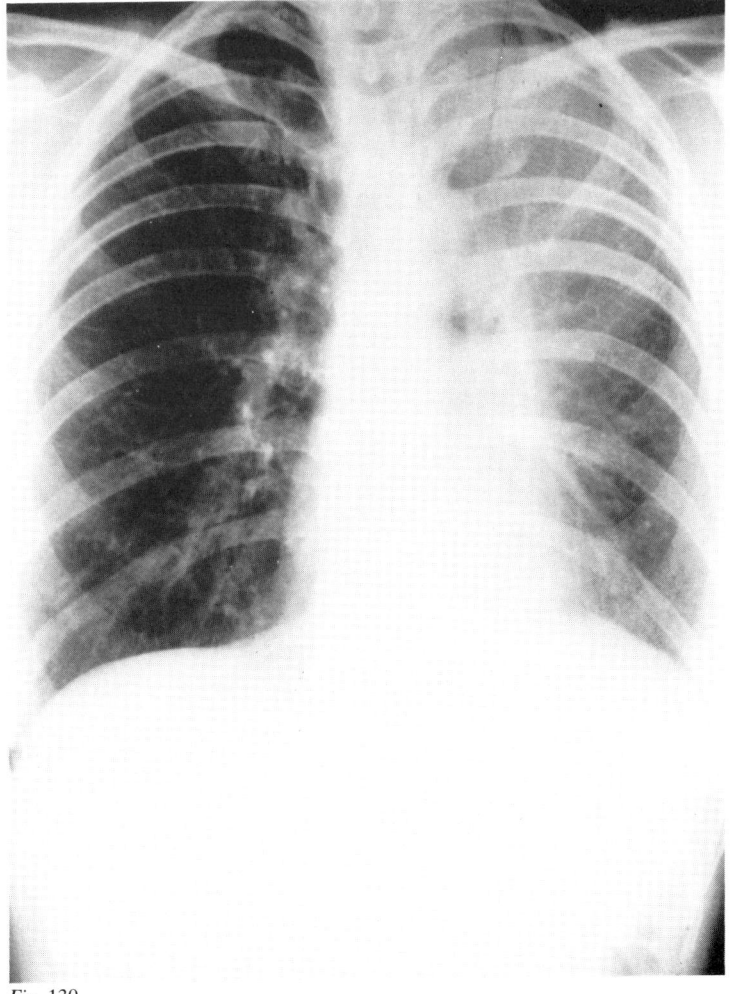

Fig. 130

Answer: Case 67

There is greater density of the left hemithorax than the right. Pulmonary vessels are visible but the left hilum and left hemidiaphragm are raised.

The appearances are those of left upper lobe collapse. This would be confirmed by a lateral film. In view of the history of asthma, mucus plugging or bronchopulmonary aspergillosis are possible causes.

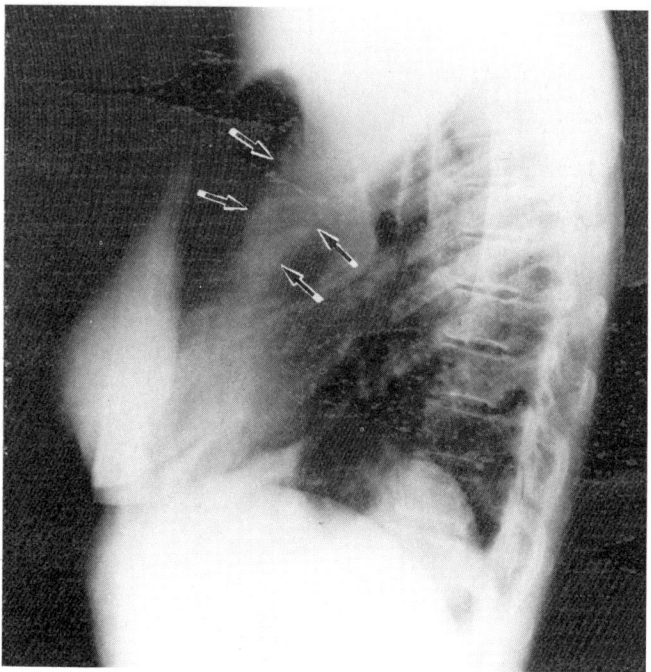

Fig. 131

Comment

The lateral film (*Fig.* 131) confirms the diagnosis of the left upper lobe collapse with the collapsed lobe shown as a 'tongue' of denser lung (arrowed).

Titres of *Aspergillus fumigatus* precipitens were very high, in keeping with bronchopulmonary aspergillosis.

Case 68

Mr Wills, aged 64, had a past history of chronic obstructive airways disease. He presented with an acute exacerbation and on examination there were widespread wheezes and coarse crackles (*Fig.* 132).

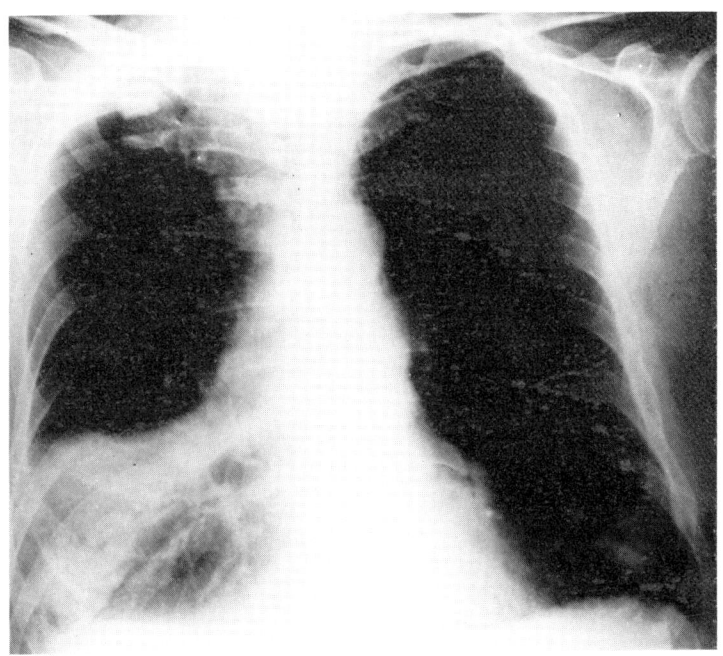

Fig. 132

Answer: Case 68

There is opacification of the right lower zone with obscuring of the right heart border. This 'silhouette sign' indicates that the opacification is adjacent to the right heart border and is thus in the right middle lobe. This is confirmed on the lateral film. (*Fig.* 133).

Within the opacified right middle lobe there is a branching pattern of translucencies—an 'air bronchogram'. This indicates that the opacity is due to opacification of the alveoli leaving the bronchi spared. This sign is most commonly seen in consolidation due to pneumonia but can occur with any fluid accumulation in the alveoli.

It can also occur as an unusual manifestation of infiltration in lymphoma and alveolar-cell carcinoma. In this case following a course of antibiotics a follow-up film showed complete resolution.

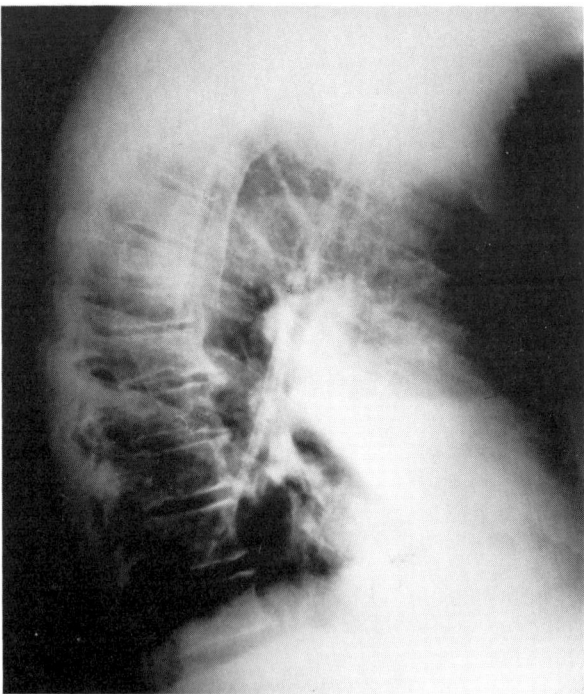

Fig. 133

Case 69

This patient had a history of bouts of dyspnoea and a productive cough. Chest X-ray and CT are shown (*Figs*. 134 and 135).

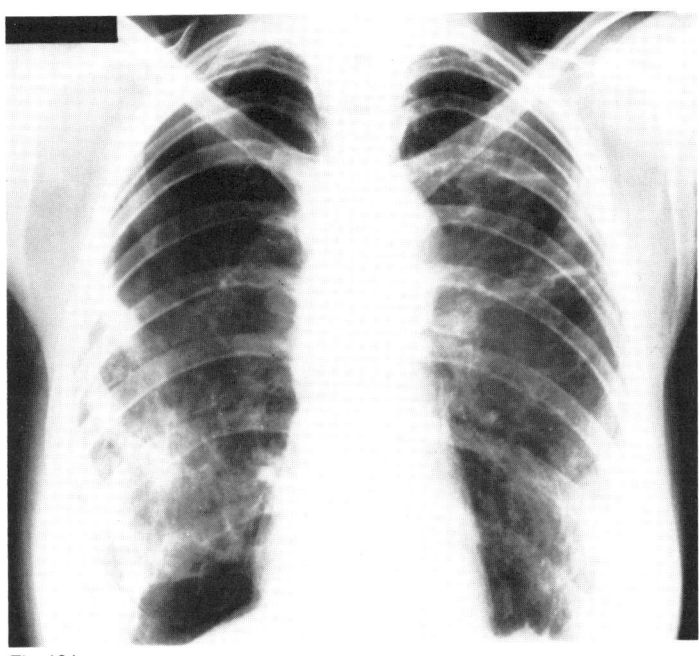

Fig. 134

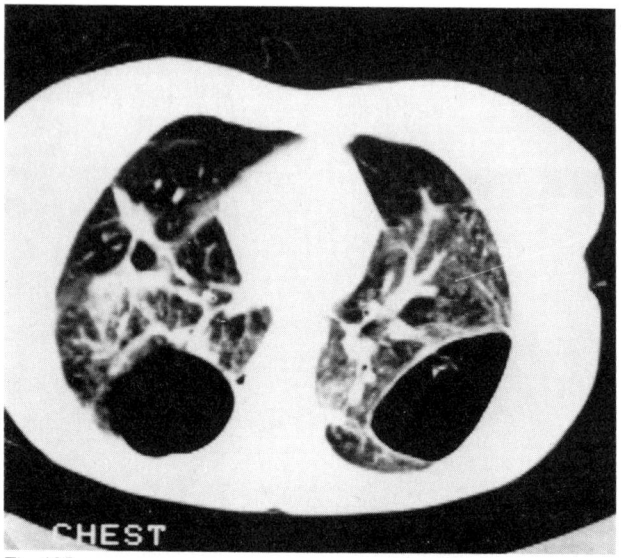

Fig. 135

Answer: Case 69

On the chest X-ray the lungs are over-expanded. There are areas of radiolucency and areas of opacification in both lungs.

The CT chest showed very large bullae throughout both lung fields but particularly affecting the periphery. There are also sheets of fibrosis and scar tissue in both lung fields.

Further Reading

Goddard, Paul R. (1987) *Diagnostic Imaging of the Chest.* London, Churchill Livingstone.

Case 70

A man, aged 60, had a painful swelling of sternum. A lateral film of the sternum and a CT scan of the chest are shown (*Figs.* 136 and 137).

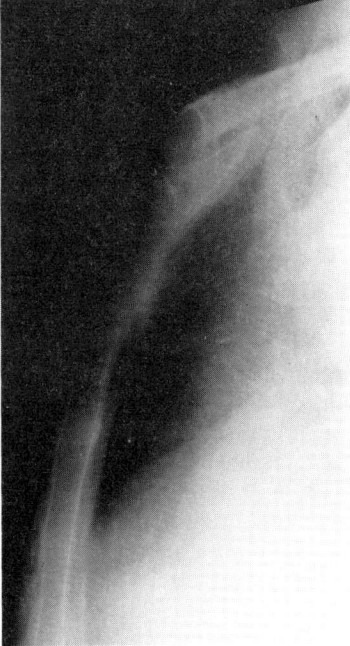

Fig. 136

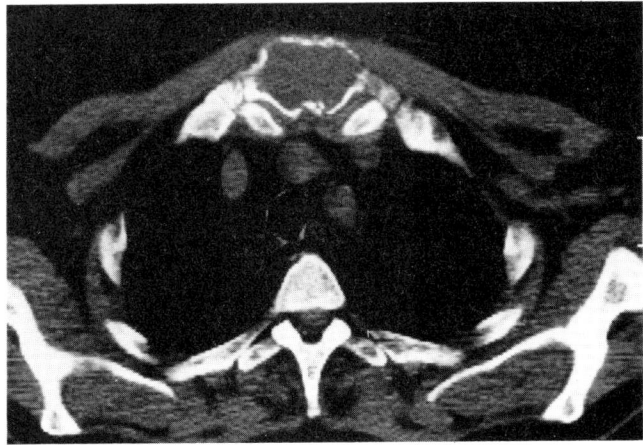

Fig. 137

Answer: Case 70

The lateral view of the sternum showed expansion of the manubrium with poor definition of the anterior margin.

The CT clearly shows a large mass of soft-tissue density centrally within the expanded manubrium with thinning and destruction of the cortex.

The appearances are thus those of a single, lytic expanding lesion in bone. Bizarre changes in the sternum, a site of adult haemopoiesis, should always arouse suspicion of a reticulosis or other haemopoietic disorder. Thus lymphoma and myeloma must be considered.

Other possible causes include metastatic carcinoma (from breast, bronchus, kidney or thyroid) giant-cell tumour and chondrosarcoma. The lack of calcification in the tumour makes chondrosarcoma less likely and this is an unusual site for giant-cell tumour.

An unusual condition which may cause a large expansile lytic lesion in bone is hydatid disease. This would, however, be a true cyst and as such would be of fluid density on CT. Other differential diagnoses to be considered are fibrous dysplasia and hyperparathyroidism. It is important to determine whether the lesion is single or multiple.

Further investigation should include a chest X-ray and blood analysis for haemoglobin and full blood count. Serum electrophoresis may reveal a monoclonal gammopathy due to myeloma. Bone scintigraphy may be useful if carcinomatous metastatic deposits are suspected.

The cause of the lesion was not revealed by these investigations. A needle biopsy of the sternum was therefore undertaken and this showed monoclonal plasma cells. The lesion was therefore a plasmacytoma. Such lesions are recognized to ultimately undergo transition to multiple myelomatosis but may remain localized for many years.

Reference

Sutton, David (1975) *Textbook of Radiology*, 2nd ed. London, Churchill Livingstone, p. 167.

Case 71

Woman, aged 52, breathless (*Fig.* 138).

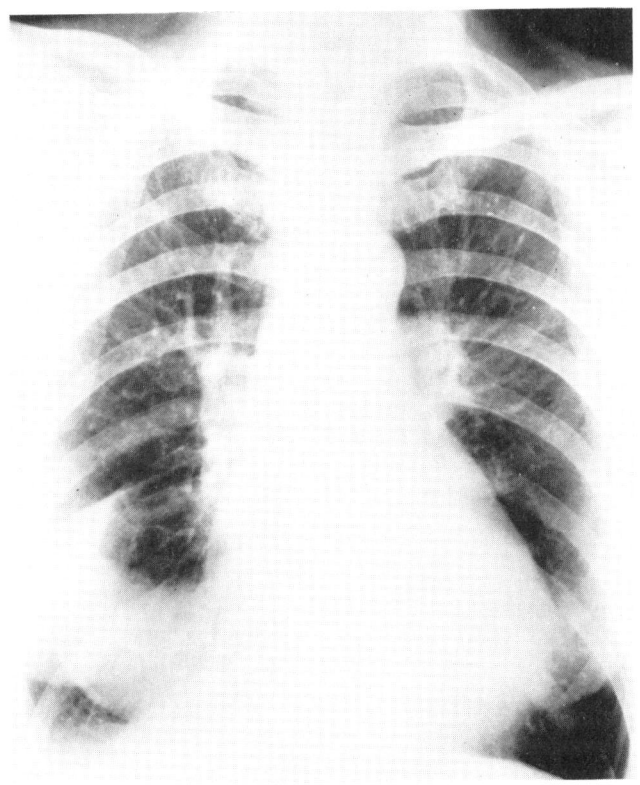

Fig. 138

Answer: Case 71

The heart is slightly enlarged and there is enlargement of the left atrial appendage. There is upper zone vessel distension.
In the right lower zone there is opacification shown to taper to a line in the superior medial edge.
There is blunting of the right costophrenic angle.
The left atrial enlargement is suggestive of mitral valve disease. In a more elderly person such appearances could be due to a variety of atrial abnormalities including ischaemia, thyrotoxicosis and amyloidosis.
The upper zone vessel distension is due to raised pulmonary venous pressure.
The right lower zone opacification is due to a pleural effusion extending into the oblique fissure, thus seen *"en face"*, and into the horizontal fissure where it is seen to taper superiorly. The patient had suffered from mitral valve disease for some years. Cardiovascular disease is covered in considerably greater detail in a companion volume in this series *"Clinical Film Viewing in Cardiovascular Disease"* by George Hartnell.

Case 72

A woman, aged 63, had a history of carcinoma of the body of the uterus treated by hysterectomy 17 years previously. She presented with the following chest X-rays (PA and lateral) (*Figs.* 139 and 140).

Case 72

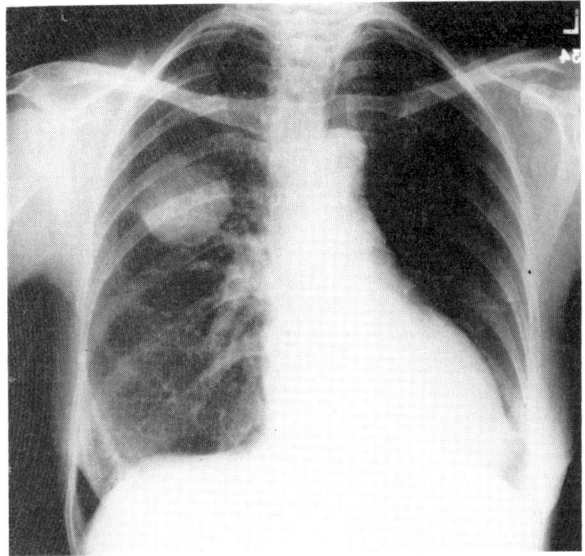

Fig. 139

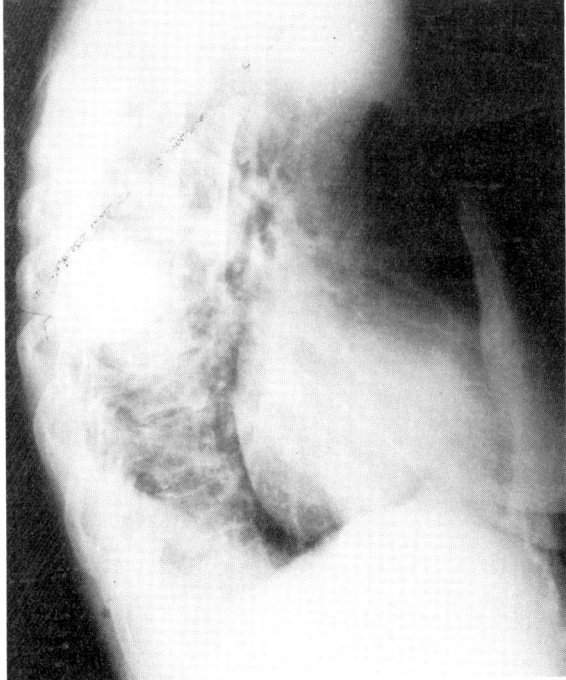

Fig. 140

Answer: Case 72

There is a large well-defined lesion in the right lung. The opacity lies in the apical segment of the right lower lobe and this is confirmed on the lateral view. There is radiolucency of the left lung field compared with the right but this is due to rotation of the patient to the left (note the asymmetry of the medial ends of the clavicles).

Serological tests showed no evidence of hydatid and the Heaf test was negative. A needle biopsy was performed under fluoroscopic control. Films are shown taken from two different projections using a rotating C-arm fluoroscopy unit (*Figs.* 141 and 142). This technique allows accurate 3-dimensional location of the needle.

Cytology of the aspirate confirmed that the mass was a secondary deposit from the carcinoma of the body of uterus.

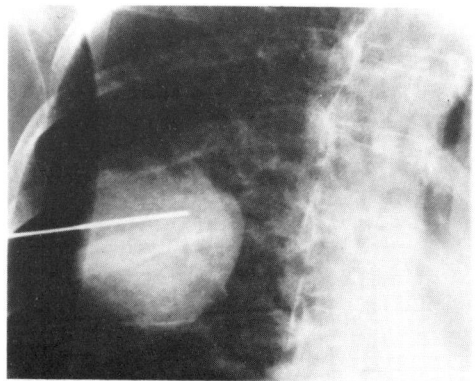

Fig. 141

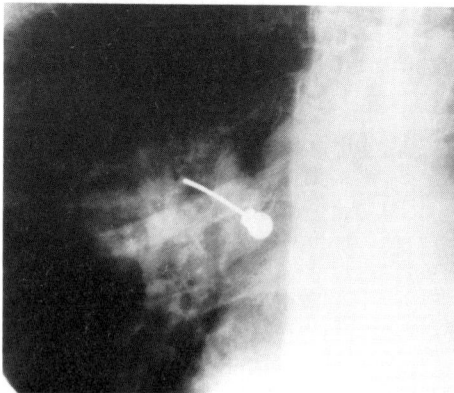

Fig. 142

Case 73

The chest X-ray of an adult female patient (*Fig.* 143)

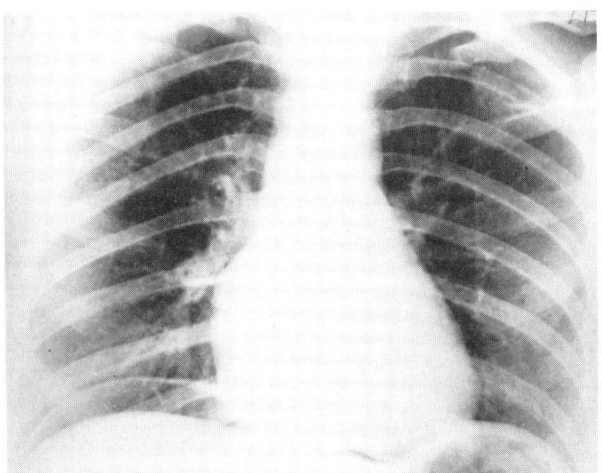

Fig. 143

Answer: Case 73

The heart and lungs are normal. There is free gas under the diaphragm, bilaterally. No other abnormality is seen.

Gas in the wrong place can get there from three sources:
1. From outside—post-laparotomy or penetrating trauma.
2. From inside—from a normally gas-containing viscus that has perforated.
3. It is made there—by gas-forming organisms (as in a subphrenic abscess).

Gas can also be wrongly diagnosed as being present under the diaphragm when it is in fact within a viscus such as the stomach or colon. The presence of free gas can be ascertained by taking a decubitus film of the abdomen. With the patient lying on her left side, a horizontal beam AP film is taken and will show free gas collected below the right abdominal wall.

In perforation the gas may only become visible after 24 hours.

Pneumoperitoneum following abdominal operations usually disappears within ten days. If present after three weeks perforation or continued leak from a hollow viscus should be suspected.

In this case there was no preceding history of trauma or surgery but a story of epigastric pain and indigestion. Laparoscopy showed a perforated duodenal ulcer.

Case 74

A farmer from Tasmania presented with the following chest X-ray. the chest X-ray and CT scan are shown (*Figs.* 144–146).

What abnormalities can be seen?

Which further investigations are suggested?

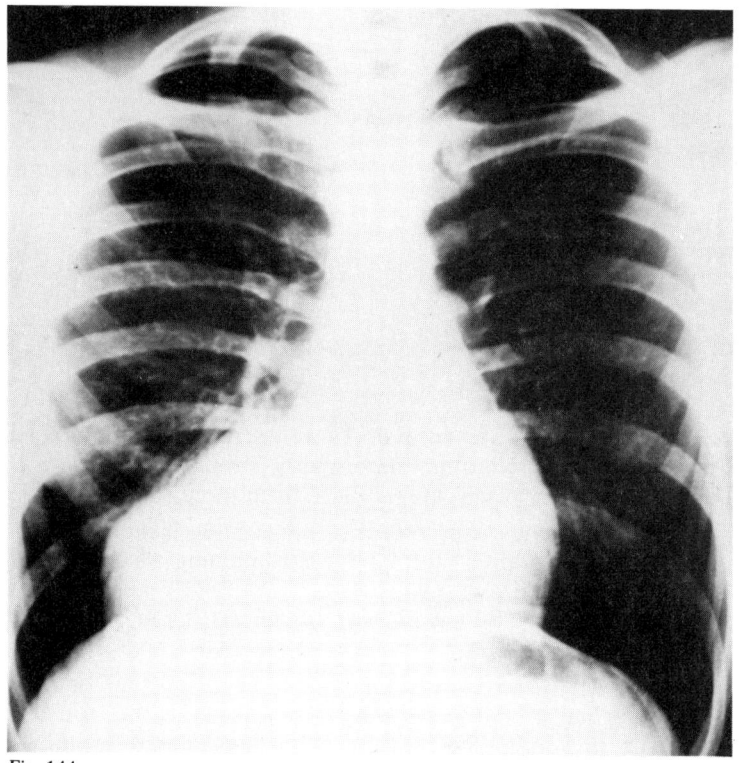

Fig. 144

Case 74

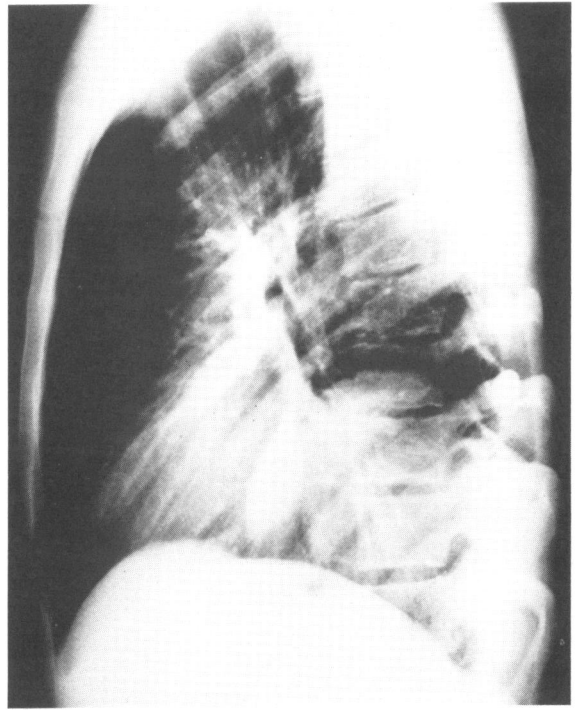

Fig. 145

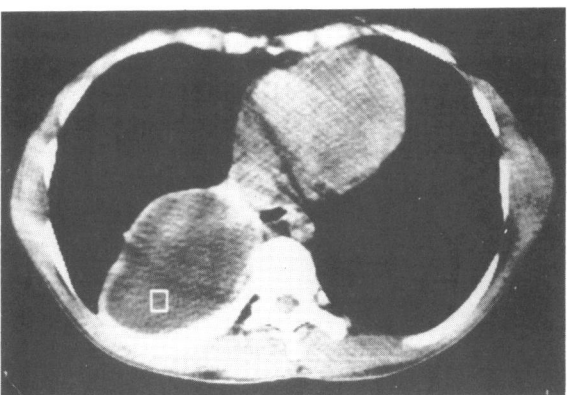

Fig. 146

Answer: Case 74

There is a large opacity in the right lower zone with obliteration of the right heart border. This is shown on the lateral film to lie posteriorly in the medial part of the right lower lobe. The mass has a very smooth outline and overlaps the cardiac outline.

CT of the chest shows a large cystic mass in the right lung (mean density 5 HU). CT of the abdomen (*Fig.* 147) shows a large cystic mass in the liver (mean density 6 HU) and a further mass containing multiple cystic lesions. The appearances are those of hydatid disease.

Hydatid disease is an infestation due to Echinococcus. This is a problem in sheep and sheepdogs. It is interesting to note that the sheep population of Tasmania is greater than the human population.

(This case is presented by courtesy of Dr Shevland.)

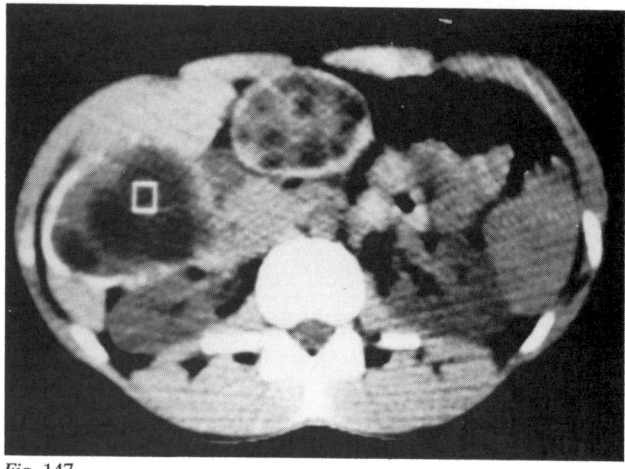

Fig. 147

Case 75

Gavin, aged 72, presented with a history of progressively worsening shortness of breath. On examination there was finger clubbing. (*Fig.* 148.)

What does the X-ray show?

How can the diagnosis be confirmed?

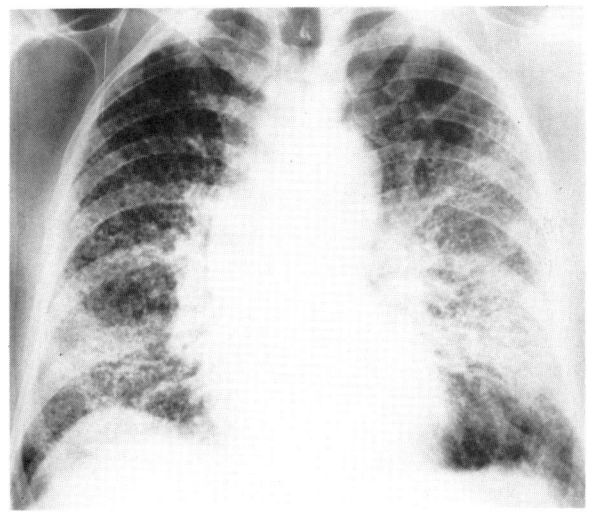

Fig. 148

Answer: Case 75

There are multiple small nodules throughout both lung fields. There are also ring shadows and lines. In view of the clinical history and presence of clubbing, cryptogenic fibrosing alveolitis is the most likely cause.

Full confirmation of the diagnosis can only be obtained by lung biopsy—either by the transbronchial route or open lung biopsy. However, a good indication of the veracity of the diagnosis can be made by computed tomography (see Case 25).

Very similar appearances can occur in fibrosing alveolitis due to rheumatoid arthritis, scleroderma, allergic alveolitides, various drug-related pneumonopathies (especially bleomycin) and cryptogenic fibrosing alveolitis. A careful history of occupation and hobbies should be obtained and blood sent for assessment of ANF and rheumatoid factor.

Case 76

A 23-year-old female patient with a known primary tumour in her right leg had the following chest X-ray and CT scans (*Figs.* 149–151).

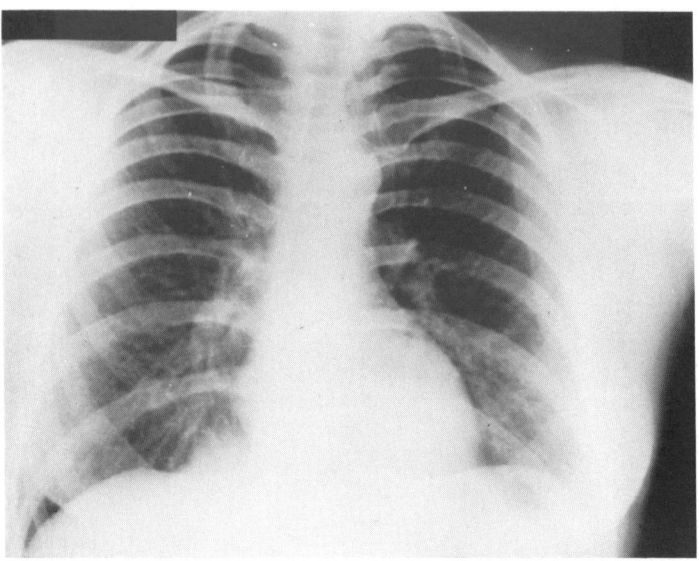

Fig. 149

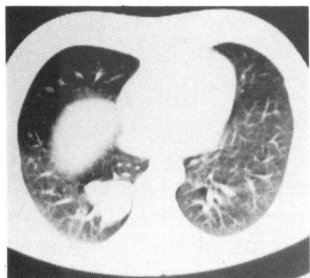

Fig. 150

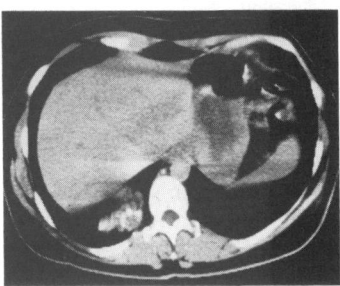

Fig. 151

Answer: Case 76

There is an opacity just visible on the chest X-ray in the right cardiophrenic angle. The CT scan shows the opacity to be well defined and partially calcified. The appearances could be due to a benign lesion, such as a tuberculoma or hamartoma, but in view of the history of a primary tumour in the leg the lesion may be an ossifying metastatic deposit from osteosarcoma.

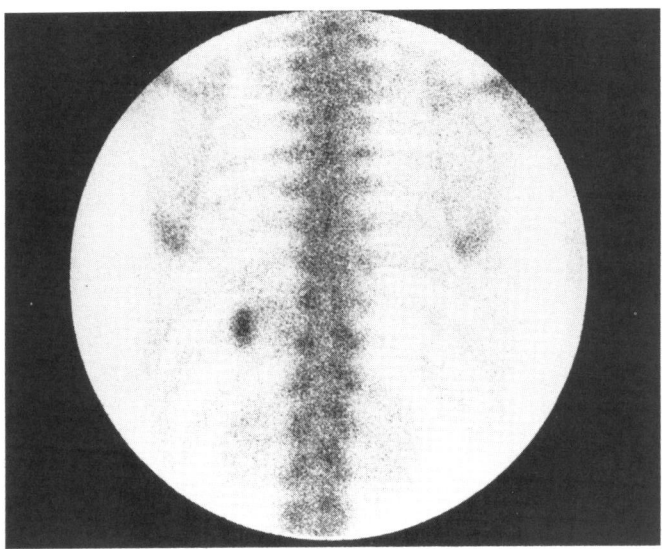

Fig. 152

Comments

A bone scan (*Fig.* 152) shows considerable uptake of radionuclide in the lesion. The patient had a primary osteosarcoma in her right femur.

Case 77

A very ill Irishman's chest X-ray (*Fig.* 153).

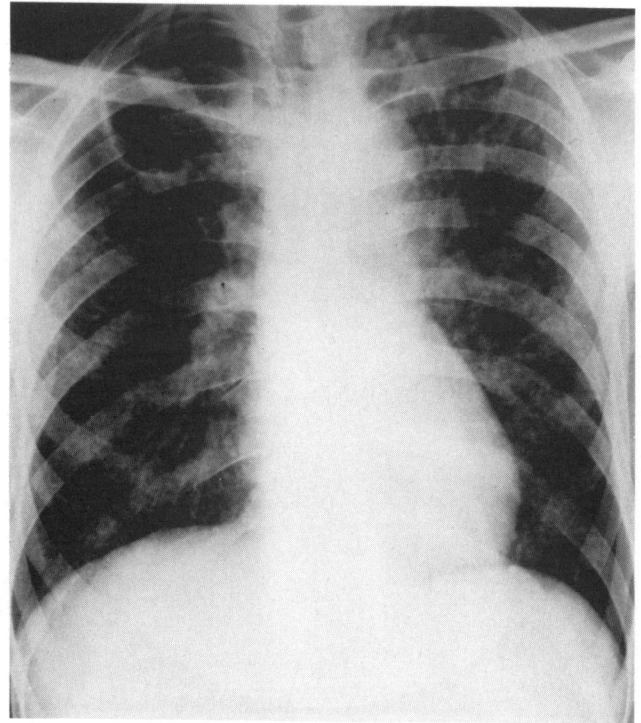

Fig. 153

Answer: Case 77

There is cavitation at both apices and widespread nodular opacities in the remainder of both lung fields. The differential diagnosis for 'miliary' nodules includes miliary tuberculosis, sarcoidosis, alveolitides (fibrosing and allergic), occupational lung diseases (pneumoconioses) and metastatic deposits..

In the presence of the cavitating apical lesions the only likely diagnosis is tuberculosis. Acid-fast bacilli were indeed present in the sputum. This is therefore a case of miliary tuberculosis complicating post-primary pulmonary tuberculosis.

Case 78

John, aged 65, had painful hands and a cough. The chest X-rays (PA and lateral) and X-ray of the hands are shown (*Figs.* 154–156).

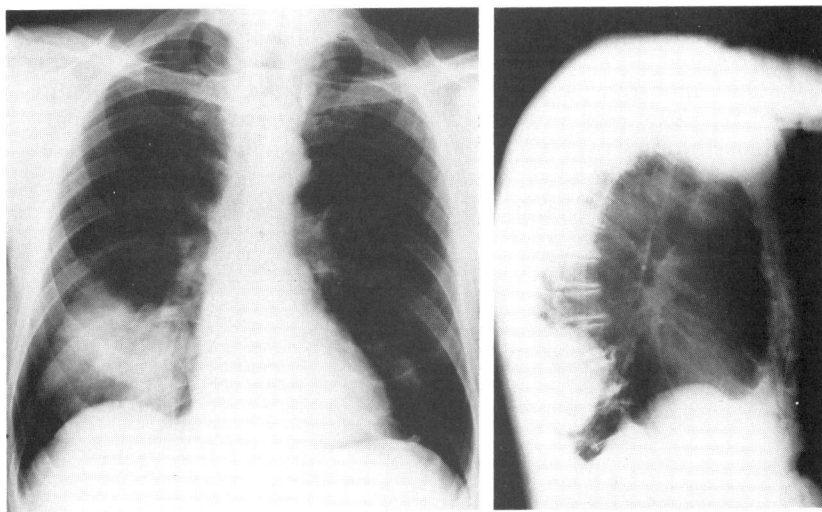

Fig. 154

Fig. 155

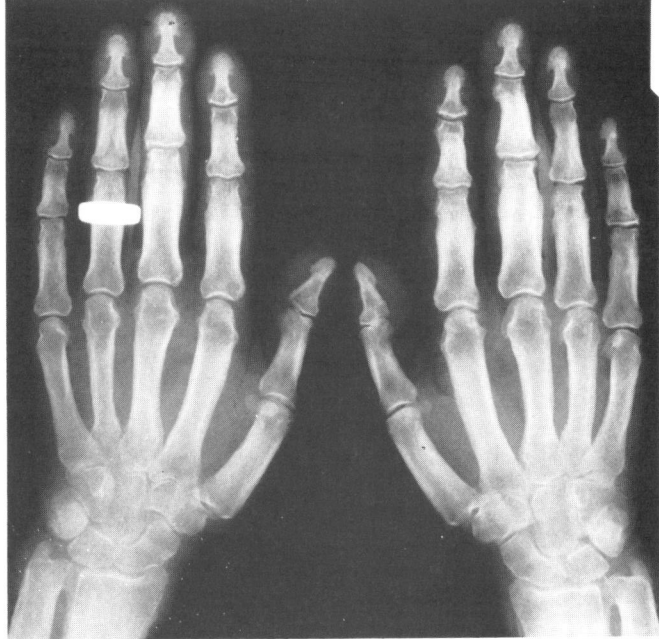

Fig. 156

Answer: Case 78

Hands

There is widespread symmetrical periosteal reaction affecting the metacarpals and proximal phalanges. The periosteal reaction is also clearly seen in the distal ends of the radii and is generally visible as a line of ossification parallel to the normal cortex.

The appearances are due to hypertrophic osteoarthropathy (HOA). This was previously known as hypertrophic pulmonary osteoarthropathy (HPOA) but recognition of non-pulmonary causes has resulted in the term 'pulmonary' being dropped from the name.

The causes of HOA are tabulated in *Table* 78.1.

Table 78.1. Causes of hypertrophic osteoarthropathy

Carcinoma of the bronchus
Pleural fibrosis
Bronchiectasis
Empyema
Cyanotic congenital heart disease
Ulcerative colitis
Cirrhosis

Similar appearances to HOA can be seen in thyroid acropachy in which the wrists and thumb are predominantly affected and 'pachydermo-periostosis' which is a familial disease associated with marked skin thickening and hyperhidrosis.

Chest

There is a large mass in the right lower lobe; CT showed this to be a single, solid mass (*Fig.* 157) and needle biopsy under fluoroscopic control (*Fig.* 158) produced a cytological diagnosis of squamous-cell carcinoma.

Carcinoma of the bronchus is by far the commonest cause of hypertrophic osteoarthropathy.

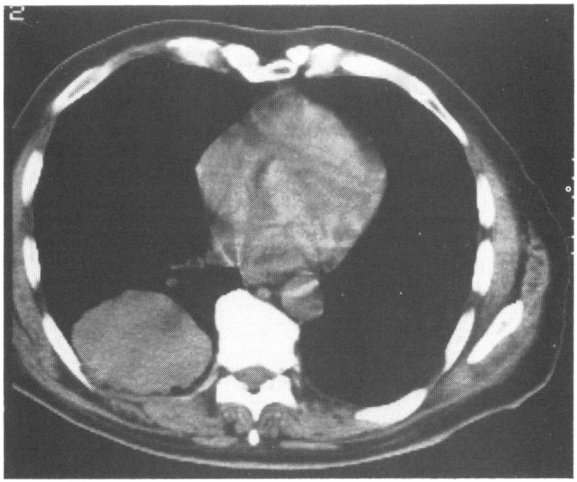

Fig. 157

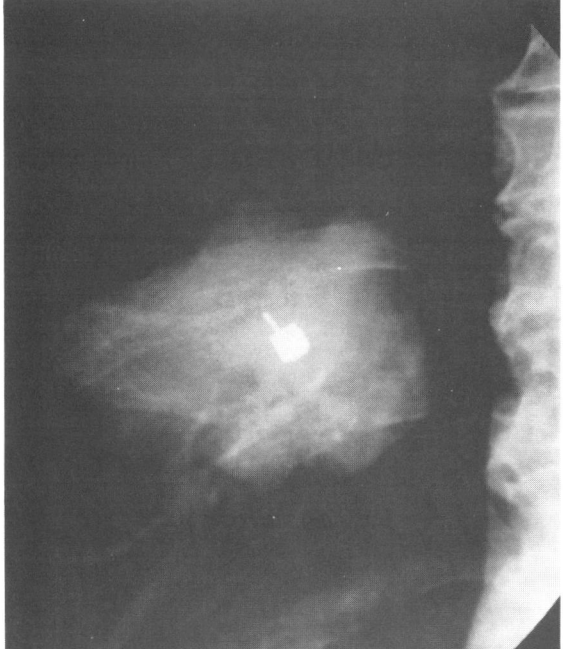

Fig. 158

Case 79

Chest X-rays (PA and lateral) and CT of a man with chronic sputum production (*Figs.* 159–162).

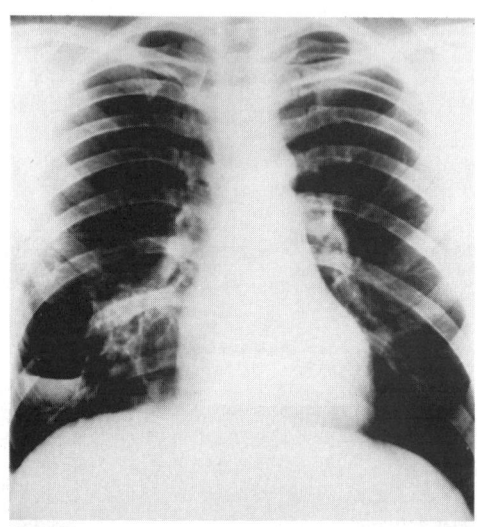

Fig. 159

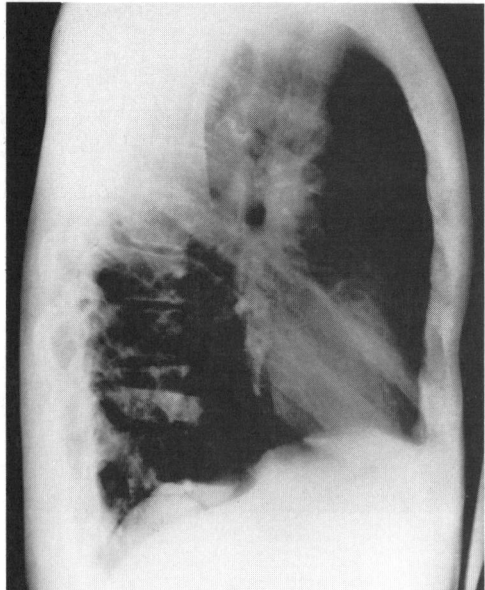

Fig. 160

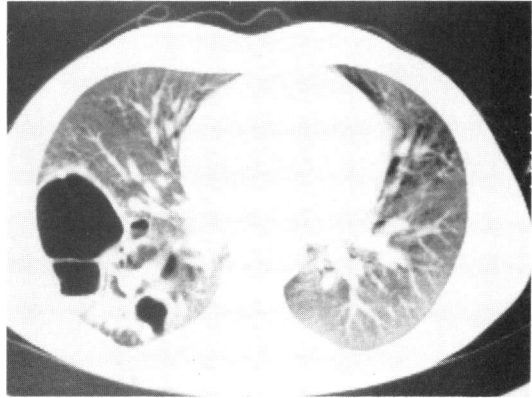

Fig. 161

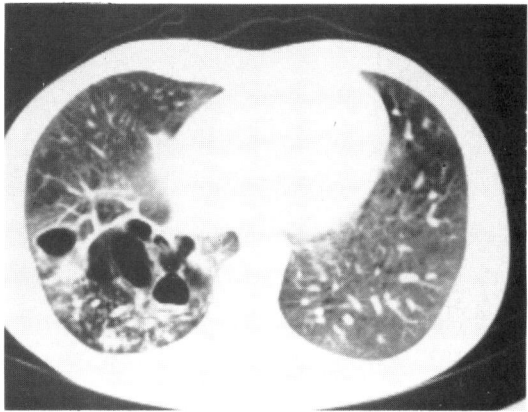

Fig. 162

Answer: Case 79

On chest PA and lateral chest a cavitating lesion is seen in the right lower zone with a definite fluid level. On the lateral film the large cavity is shown posteriority

On CT chest multiple cavities are seen adjacent to blood vessels. The appearances are those of bronchocoeles due to bronchiectasis. The abnormality is confined to the right lower lobe and the patient may well benefit from surgery.

Comment

This case should be compared with Case 69 in which bullae are seen peripherally

Case 80

Charlotte, aged 79, had progressively developing weakness in her legs.

Her chest X-ray and magnetic resonance imaging (MRI) scan of cervical and thoracic spine are shown (T1 weighted scan, Picker Vista 0.5T) (*Figs.* 163 and 164).

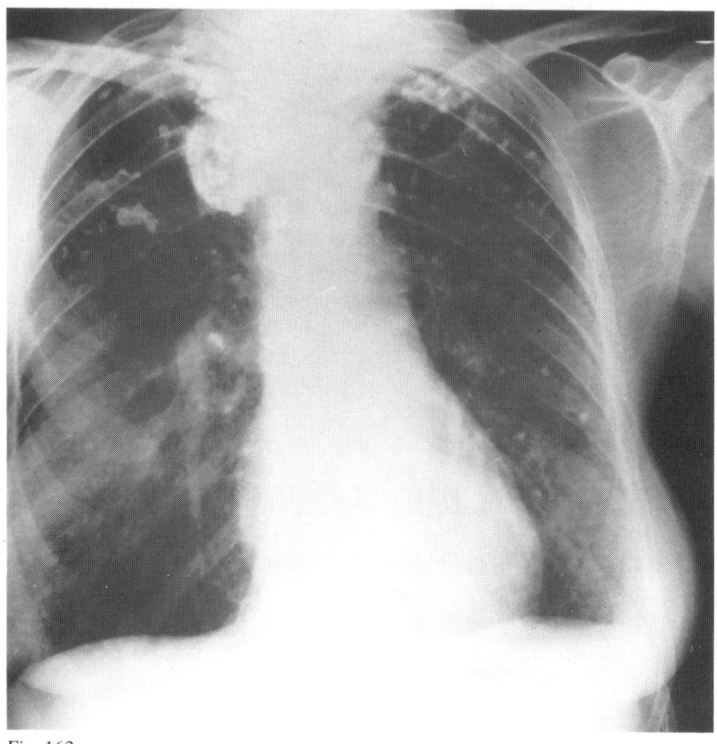

Fig. 163

Case 80

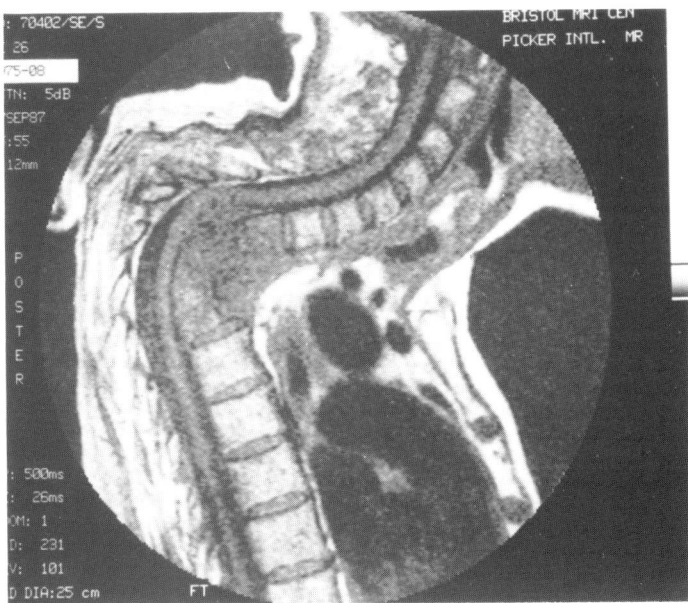

Fig. 164

Answer: Case 80

On the chest X-ray there is calcification in the apices and in the mediastinum. The appearances are consistent with old tuberculosis.

On MRI of the spine there is destruction of T1 to T4 vertebral bodies and intervertebral discs. There is a soft-tissue mass anteriorly and posteriorly to the vertebral bodies with compression of the spinal cord. There is marked angulation of the spine.

The appearances are those of tuberculous spondylitis.

Comment

The spinal cord was decompressed surgically with good effect. Tuberculosis was confirmed and treated with antituberculous chemotherapy.

Magnetic resonance imaging is covered in two forthcoming books to be published by Clinical Press (*An Introduction to Clinical MRI* and *Film Viewing in CT and MRI*).

(MRI scans by courtesy of Bristol MRI Centre.)

■ Index

Note: The subject may be referred to in the Question or Answer section or in both. The numbers refer to case numbers and not to the page number.

Alpha-l-antiprotease (antitrypsin) deficiency 45
Abscess, pulmonary 17
Achalasia 3
Actinomycosis 60
Adult Respiratory Distress Syndrome 16
Agenesis 12
AIDS 16, 28
Air bronchogram 17, 28, 68
Air in the wrong place, table of causes 27
Allergic alveolitis 54
Alveolar opacification 5, 28, 53
Alveolar opacification, table of causes 28
Aneurysm 1
Aneurysm traumatic 4
Aneurysm, syphilitic 61
Arterio-venous malformation 32
Arteriography 4
Asbestos exposure 47, 49, 61, 65
Aspergillus fumigatus 21
Asthma 14, 67

'Bird-fancier's lung' 54
Bochdalek hernia 2
Bronchiectasis 79
Broncho-pulmonary aspergillosis 21, 67
Bronchocoele 79
Bronchogenic cyst 2

Calcified pulmonary mass 31
Carcinoma of the breast 24
Carcinoma of the bronchus 11, 13, 15, 18, 29, 63, 78
Cavitation, pulmonary 17
Cervical ribs 37
Chest pain 1
Co-arctation of the aorta 36
Collapse, left lower lobe 16
Collapse, left upper lobe 15, 67
Collapse, right middle lobe 14
Collapse, right upper lobe 13
Computed tomography 1, 7, 11, 18, 20, 21, 25, 29, 57, 60, 61, 62, 69, 70, 76, 78, 79

Computed tomography, needle biopsy 29
Consolidation, right middle lobe 16
Contusion 7, 8

Deep vein thrombosis 44
Diaphragm, raised 6, 8, 41, 64
Diaphragm, rupture 6, 64
Dissecting aneurysm 1

Echinococcus granulosus 30, 74
Effusion, encysted 33
Emphysema 45, 69
Emphysema, obstructive 43
Emphysema, surgical 8
Empyema 46
Encysted effusion 33, 71
Eventration of the diaphragm 41

Fat Embolism 5
Fibrosing alveolitis 25, 62, 75

Gastric pull-through 60
Goodpasture's syndrome 53

Haemothorax 7, 8
Hilar enlargement, table of causes 9
Hilum, increased density 11
Hodgkin's lymphoma 2, 20
Hyaline membrane disease 52
Hyatid cyst 30, 74
Hypertrophic osteoarthropathy 78
Hypertrophic osteoarthropathy, table of causes 78
Hypoplasia 12

Increased bone density, table of casues 35
Infarction 16
Infectious mononucleosis 56
Inhaled peanut 43

Index

Left lower lobe collapse 16
Left upper lobe collapse 15, 67
Leukaemia 28
Lipoma, pleural 49
Lymphangitis carcinomatosa 24

Magnetic resonance imaging 56, 80
Mastectomy 24, 42
Mediastinal mass, table of causes 2
Mediastinal mass flowchart 1
Mediastinal widening 1, 2, 3, 4, 11
Microlithiasis alveolaris 26
Miliary nodularity 22–26
Miliary nodularity, table of causes 22
Miliary nodularity in, childhood, table of causes 54
Miliary nodularity, high density, table of causes 26
Miliary tuberculosis 22, 77
Mycetoma 21
Myeloma 70

Needle biopsy 29, 72, 78
Non-resolving consolidation, table of causes 16

Obstructive emphysema 43
Opacification of a hemithorax, table of causes 12
Oesophageal carcinoma 59
Osteosarcoma 76

Paediatric chest problems 51–56
Pancoast tumour 18
Paraspinal masses, table of causes 39
Pectus excavatum 38
Pharyngeal pouch 2
Plasmacytoma 70
Pleural based opacity 46
Pleural based opacity, table of causes 46
Pleural effusion asbestos, exposure 47
Pleural plaques 49, 65
Pneumoconiosis 23, 58
Pneumocystis pneumonia 28
Pneumoperitoneum 27, 73
Pneumothorax 51, 63
Progressive massive fibrosis 23, 58
Pulmonary arterial, hypertension 40
Pulmonary cavitation 17, 18, 19, 20, 21

Pulmonary embolism 7, 44
Pulmonary opacity, flowchart 29

Raised hemidiaphragm 6, 8
Respiratory distress syndrome, of the newborn 52
Respiratory distress in the newborn, table of causes 15
Ribs: expansile lesions 35
Rib fractures 6, 8
Rib notching, table of causes 36
Ribs: sclerotic 34
Right middle lobe collapse 14
Right middle lobe consolidation 16
Right upper lobe collapse 13
Ruptured aorta 4
Ruptured diaphragm 6

Sarcoidosis 2, 9, 66
Silhouette sign 14, 16, 68
Staphylococcal abscess 17
Subdural haematoma 7
Superior vena cava, obstruction 11
Surgical emphysema 8
Syphilitic aortitis 61

Thymoma 2
Thyroid goitre 2, 58
Trauma 4, 5, 6, 7, 8, 64
Tuberculoma 31
Tuberculosis 27
Tuberculosis, chest wall 50
Tuberculosis, miliary 22, 77
Tuberculosis, primary 10
Tuberculosis, spinal 39, 80

Unilateral translucency 42
Unilateral translucency, table of causes 42

Venography 44
Ventilation/Perfusion studies 7, 44, 48

Wegener's granulomatosis 19
Wilm's tumour 55